T0062517

# MENTAL ILLNESS, BIPOLAR AND RACISM

VOLUME 2

ANEB JAH RASTA SENSAS-UTCHA NEFER I

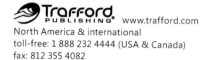
www.trafford.com
North America & international
toll-free: 1 888 232 4444 (USA & Canada)
fax: 812 355 4082

**M**ental Illness is of various illnesses that are physiological, hereditary and environmental. In this, bipolar has been an epidemic from the creation and origins of the universe. Through electromagnetic and neurotransmitters of the human anatomy, this is specified within every sense of the body of an organism. Within the body of an organism, there are millions of frequencies of neuro-waves and electromagnetic forces that are used and serve as forms transmissions within every single life-force. Therefore, cognitively, behaviors are often triggered by patterns and wavelengths that are within the central nervous system, peripheral nervous system as well as the anatomical nervous system. In this, there are ancestral plasmas that are caused by diseases that have occurred throughout an individual's family tree. This is through the genes of the individual where we find the individual purpose for being a part of the universal origin of the Tree of Life.

Therefore, we must understand that there are many cases and stages that one must overcome and overtake. In this, there has to be a crucifixion of one's person. Meaning, there has to be a death of the flesh and a much greater growth and development of the individual's spirit. In dying to our person, we must first come to the realization that we are in the image and essence of God. As written in all religions, god is the main objective. However the subjective realms reveal the purpose and destiny of ones path for seeking and pursuing God.

In this, mental illness has shaped all human factors of discipline. This is from western medicine, religion, theology as well as philosophy. This is by all means and understandings that The Shemites and Japhites aren't the individuals who have been ordained to rule mankind as written in The King James version of the Bible. In 1611, when the King James Version of the Bible was written, all of its scholars were of the Caucasian race. Therefore, we all know that there has to be some misunderstandings. Those misconceptions have imprisoned humanity for multitudes of generations. Therefore, generations and nations; especially the Black race have been disenfranchised from the origins of western thought.

Racism is mental illness and bipolar. The mechanism of bipolar mania has various stages of mania and suicidal tendencies. In saying this, there has to be some kind of solution. That solution is to develop the understanding of one's self. I am not talking about self-centeredness nor self-righteousness. I am informing you, the reader; that there must be a solution of and a shaping of your spiritual and religious knowledge and understanding. In doing this, you must study all forms of science, theology, psychology and medicine. In doing so, you'll grasp a greater knowledge and understanding as you have meditated on this in the Khamitic science. This will enable you to recognize the qualities and inequalities of you true self. As, your true self dies you'll be empowered with the powers of God.

Qualities of God is what you'll have. Therefore, you must work out your own salvation as the bible says. However, you must have a strong appetite for the love, understanding and wisdom of God. For God is inside of all living organisms. Therefore, beware of the schemers. For they too have knowledge of who God is. However, they only want to work on the unstable individuals in order to attain the wealth of the economical and western man! They are sahu in nature. Those individuals are only there—in your life to gain your assets and steal your divinity. However, by recognizing that you are a god; you'll begin to notice their purpose as well as your own. Life a simple and pleasurable. Therefore, live to the fullest.

Meditation and trance are within reach. Within reach, we shall seek and find answers that have been hidden by mankind from the origins of The King James Version of The Bible. Now, within the Quran, that's another subject to be discussed another time later. However, within the Quran as well as all other forms of religion; it is assumed the Egypt is polytheistic. However, Khamit is a monotheistic culture that studies several attributes of one God Ausar! Therefore; what is really the Tree of Knowledge of Good and Evil! You see, for generations, individuals have lost their minds as a result of failing to grasp the understanding of the entire Tree of Life. However, they study the Yoruba and Hebrew doctrine that are within The Bible. They lack the understanding that they too had gotten their knowledge and understanding from ancient Egypt. In addition, they call it a pagan society. Western religions are loquacious, murderers, thieves, omnivores and cannibals. As they read their bibles, they are denouncing and fooling themselves. Satan is divided within itself. So is its kingdom too divided within.

In this volume 2 of Mental Illness / Bipolar, you, the reader will receive an awakened soul as well as spirit. You'll have a restructured and motivated spirit. So, get off of your lazy ass. Do something positive for someone and self. In addition, millions of individuals with bipolar and other mental disabilities seem to sit on their pity and feel that they are exceptions to being disciplined. They too must also comprehend the nature of their disability and not use this as a free-for-all form of ceremonial advocacy for their inheritance of disability benefits as well as other forms of benefits that comes along with this. Moreover, a mental disability is not the cause of one being a schemer, cheater, liar and or thief. However, these individuals often make excuses for their disability by uses and abuses of narcotics and alcoholic beverages. This also involves the over indulging and manipulation through sexual perversions and extreme acts of immoral.

You see, some are often apologetic and are at ease when scapegoats. In this, they often say that their depression has caused them to behave a certain a certain way or certain ways. Truly, they need spiritual growth, development and nurturing in all areas of their lives as well as every person on the face of the earth. Whatsoever a person think he or she is he or she shall then become. Because the nature and power of the tongue is powerful. Therefore, these are considered words of power. In addition, healing has no place in the lives of most people due to their conditioned and westernized ways of living, thinking, speaking and lifestyle. This is characterized by bipolar and its livings processes. In this, energy is then generated by electrical current and magnetic forces of the spirit and later transferred unto mankind. There are various unseen factors of the spirit. Unseen factors and forces are considered to be difficult to recognize by the human eye. You see, we are all images and in the likeness of God! We were created form love. Love is healing! Love is understanding. And Love of the power of God!

Finally, in this book, you'll get an understanding of where you fit in the puzzle of the hierarchy of life. Life of which God has preordained for you. This is in order for you to live a prosperous life by being delivered from your infirmities and strongholds. These have kept you beneath your destiny and fulfilling your life in being one with your god as well as the Creator of all things. Are you ready to grow and become what you have not known. Do you recognize that your own abilities cannot change and improve your behaviour. Are you calling on God or Pagans? Healing comes from the powers that are within. Are you healing?

You will have an understanding of your healing progression when you realize that there's an important medical issue that is disharmonizing your spirit. In this, the mental health act of the United States of America has been established to assist those who are in need of assistance, meaning those who are incapable of working and those who are in need of financial assistance. However; millions of individuals have manipulated the system as well as others with spiritual wickedness. They have been clever in many ways of scheming and scandal. In this, they have committed various forms of satanic ritual on themselves and others due to their cheating, lying and denying behaviors of Westernized thought and religion. You see, an individual with a mental illness has to first recognize that there's a problem with his or her nervous systems. Secondly, the individual with a mental illness must seek to find out what the various problems are that he or she is having.

Thirdly, this particular individual mustn't be in denial—admit that there is a health issue. Finally, get the needed assistance.

In this; they call this organizational assistance and or "circle-of friends"! This means that your circle of friends shall not manipulate one's self, peers and or the system. This is done by scoffing and tapping into one's future in order to impede the progress of another. They rob you from yourself if you haven't recognized their spiritual cleverness. Their cleverness is to materialize and demonize your every form of progression. Their hypocritical motives and behaviors will seduce the lower portion your spirit-soul and being. This leaves individuals hopeless in their quest into becoming the essence of God. Thieves will capture you by seducing you into their abominable desires of spiritual and mental slavery.

This is the setian spirit and personality of the western man. As the western man does. As western theology has taught and programmed the world ever since and prior to the bible being written. This has been brought throughout many generations of the world. You cannot be a manipulator and serve God too by using survival techniques to tame and control another's next and every intention through the lower self of another. Individuals go into prayer {fault-finding} people to impede through envy and not for the love of God. Prayer doesn't heal the issue. This is a behaviour and a spiritual condition of the lower man. You see, people will talk to you by discussing parables surrounding your life if you aren't aware of yourself. They have fooled you in the sense of sahuism. That is what the church does as well as witches and devils. This is criminal and shameful. Criminal and shameful by the means of the setian forces of psychosis.

This is Utchau Metu! The weighing of words in a universal form of awareness. By catching the Rat and poisoning it. They steal your blessings. The seduce you into their misleading forms of God! The lower part of your being is seduced as written in the Metu Neter Volume 1. Indeed there are scoffers who are waiting to steal and enslave you mentally. Yes, mental illness is the variation of several illnesses that is caused by ancestral disorders. This deals with modernity and futuristic forms of prophesy that has to be fulfilled in your life. Don't let the setians get you. Therefore, work on your own spiritual development. However, setians fail to work on their own spiritual development. Therefore, there's no healing within them. They seek outside sources and forces for healing-information doesn't heal. You see; I can teach and preach to you people. However, if you aren't looking up you'll die in eternal damnation. You people seek a god for healing. However, you fail to follow HIS principles of meditation, diet and exercise.

In addition; prayer is defined as the following; an invocation or act that begins to activate a rapport with a deity, an object of worship or a spiritual entity through deliberate communication. Therefore, in western theology and philosophy—it states that there shouldn't be long prayers Mark 12:40 as Jesus states. Matthew 11:30 "my yoke is easy"—"take on my burdens"! Moreover, the definition of yoke is as follows; something that causes people to be treated with cruelty and unfairly by taking away their freedom. Yoke is also a wooden frame or bar that is used to join things; such as animals, spirits and people. They are joined at the head and or neck for working together by force. This too is racism, criminal and mental slavery! Therefore, if your yoke is easy and prayer invokes a deity or spiritual being—individuals become mentally impaired by force and or invocation. This is negative karma! For they seduce unstable souls as written in the epistle of Peter—which too is out of Greece. Greece is a Caucasian ad Arab nation of the people of Shem and Japheth. In addition, those that are suffering from mental illnesses too are negligent for committing grave forms of idolatry through manipulation.

Deuteronomy 28:28 The lord, their leader, pastor or priest shall smite thee with madness of the mind and blindness with astonishment of the heart. In the concordance it says "the lord will smite you with blindness and confusion of the mind! Deuteronomy 28:65 says "the lord will give you an anxious mind. Now this is what the bible says. Who wrote it! This is racism and hatred. Therefore; King Saul of Tarsus, who later became Paul after committing suicide, wrote to the people of Gaul the following; Oh, foolish Galatians"—"who bewitched you"! This is the deceptiveness of Paul who was King Saul during King David's reign.

Moving right along. The word bewitched means to enchant someone by fascination; to be very desirable to someone, to cast a spell on someone, to affect someone or something by using a magical spell. People believe that the opposite sex has been fascinated with and or by them by attraction or delight in way that seems to be magical. Also, to make someone say, think or do something by putting under a spell. The listed is invocation prayer by seeking others to respond to their authority by excluding God. This is because, you are oneness, in the image and likeness of God as written in the book of Genesis as Eastern spirituality teaches verses the western forms. You see, everyone has agreed with that of the European Race in committing falsehoods against ancient Egypt. They will continue to deceive helpless individuals. This too is occurring in the church. They are casting spells on individuals without understanding the Word of God. Which is the Metu Neter Oracle! You see, this is mentioned in The Schizophrenic Black Church of The Jihad. This confirms my claim against the church. Deuteronomy 18: 10-12 they call up omens by calling up the dead which is forbidden. They call up Jesus to save them which he forbade in Mark 12:40. Christianity is hypocritical. Western Religion is hypocritical. Whenever the truth arrives, they're in denial; this leads to a grave form of mental illness. This is crazy and scary to you. Yet, it is the spiritual truth. As one says "you can't have your cake and eat it"! Jesus wasn't a Christian! He was a Hebrew. You see, Hebrews study the Kabballah of which they got from ancient Egypt! Hebrews 4: 12-14 the word of God is quick and powerful, and sharper than a two-edged sword and cleansing of the soul, spirit and of the joints marrow. Marrow is the inner cavity of the bones that is a major site of blood cell production! Therefore, mental illness / bipolar is of various conditions characterized by impairment of an individual's normal cognitive, emotional and behavioral functioning. This is caused by ancestral pathogens and curses through heredity and genetics. In this, there are several to discerning the spirit and healing. However, individuals has wasted valuable time by the consumption information through the lower forms of khaibet level of the Tree of Life Meditation System. Many individuals will not heal due to arrogance and ignorance. Deuteronomy 28:61 you'll have diseases that aren't in this book and you will not be cured. Continue to read your bibles and deny the truth. You see, western man will often select a feel-good approach in forgiveness and healing. They select certain deities by force and enchantment without having them within their presence. The Metu Neter Oracle is not a fortunetelling device. It is for spiritual growth and development. King Saul persuaded the witch of Endor to bring out Samuel. That is omenism. This was a practice of which he once forbade. God sees all hidden this. God knows all of your ways and thoughts prior to committing them. You are fooling yourselves by reading horoscopes daily. That has nothing at to do with spirituality and healing. That is a quick fix, a satanic device. 2 Corinthians 2:11. That is why you'll have mental breakdowns and delusions of the flesh and of the spirit. You'll have a warped persona & spirit. 1 Timothy 4:1-3. This is the doctrine of devils. For they promise you liberty; for whom a man is overcome; the same is he who is brought into the bondage of mental and physical slavery. Therefore; choose whom you shall serve. As Joshua lied, robbed and conquered the Canaanites he said "Choose Whom You Shall Serve"! Joshua 24:15. This is the curse of Canaan and Ham of which ancient Egypt once reigned. Egypt was a class civilization prior to it being invaded and raided by the Jews, Hebrews, Arabs and Caucasians through the preordained forms of yoking. Egypt is the creator of religion, medicine and spirituality.

In this, Jesus changed Apostle Peter's name to Simon-Peter during the denial by Peter to him. Peter denied Jesus three time as written in the gospels. In addition, 1 Peter 5:8 Be alert and of sober mind. Your enemy the devil prowls around like a roaring lion looking for someone to devour. Now! Who is the so-called Lion of The Tribe of Judah! That's another story within itself. Therefore; James 2:2 Beware of personal favoritism. Whereas; individuals often say that they are favored by the Most High God! Their Lord and Savior Jesus Christ. However, if your westernized scripture says there is to be no personal favoritism—then why are you worshipping a polytheistic deity in Jesus-Christ? Christ won't save you! Everyone is born in the image and likeness of God. We are of God! You are a god.

James 2:2 suppose a man comes to your meeting a gold ring and fine clothing and a poor man comes to you wearing filthy clothing also comes in; and you show special attention to the man wearing fine clothing and you say to the man well dressed "here's a good seat for you". But say to the poor man, "sit at my feet". You see that is racism in a nutshell. Therefore; had you not discriminated amongst yourselves! And become judges with evil thoughts. This is the same with God. Segregation of the western religious doctrines have dismantled the human race for millions of centuries. Once again, Jesus was a Hebrew a non-Christian. This controversy is also a part of the mental health act and civil rights acts that forbids discriminatory actions against anyone—for any purpose. Again, inclusion, circle of friends and so forth and so on! Discrimination, the Ausarian religion is monotheistic and believes in various attributes of one god. However, on the other hand; Christianity is polytheistic which believes in many such as; the Christ, Jesus, the Father, Son and Holy Ghost. This is extremely the goal of the setian and his wickedness of mind control and universal mental slavery. This is also mentioned in the Quran. Therefore; stop fooling others with this fallacious form of Shakespearianism, ignorance, arrogance, defiance, treachery as well as slavery.

# DO YOUR PART

This writing is not out Greece. However 1 Corinthians 3:2 I fed you with milk and not solid food. For you weren't ready for it. Therefore; you understood not. Indeed, you are still not ready for God's word, The Metu Neter Oracle. Therefore, bringing out the past, meaning where you were prior to gaining an understanding of this sound doctrine before you became an Ausarian by resurrection of the Ausarian Religion. You must awaken the spiritual mantra of Sebek. This specific mantra allows one to positively segregate and logically weight all decisions and judgments through the mantra of Maat. In addition, you will notice by seeing your hidden enemies through the Nekhebet and Uatchet mantras of receptivity. You are capable of dwelling amongst your enemies through the powers of Amen.

In addition, the Ausarian religion lives on a vegan diet. This a non-dairy and non-omnivorous diet. We are herbivores. We eat no meats. Yet, dairy substitutes as well as whole grains, fruits and vegetables. This diet allows us to reduce vitamin and nutrient deficiencies that will eventually lead to greater forms of physiological and chronic illnesses. You see, the Khametic culture recognizes that diseases and illness stem from lack of exercise, alcohol and drug dependency and eating habits that are poor. Their factors coincide with the westernized spiritual attitude. In this, stress is chronic. It worsens in individuals that are having to deal with their spiritual depravation. Their depravation has caused them to remain at the lower of the left hemisphere of the brain. This is the sahu man. The logical and syllogistic creature that is searching for means of survival instead recognizing the underlying problems of his or her own health. Healing is the manifestation of Gods' power and authority. Do you want to become a god? You have the power. You have the power to be free from disease and disability. Hope is only a word used to relieve hostility. Therefore; you must do your part by meditation, diet and exercise. People, stop making excuses. Work out your own salvation. Healing is only the first step to a new life. A new life only empowers one to overcome every single obstacle that has hindered one's spiritual development.

God. God intended for mankind to have dominion over all things. Therefore, in dominion, I ask that you comprehend the Tree of Life Meditation System by Ra Un Nefer Amen. You see, life is a spectrum of fulfillment and infinite prophetic wisdom. In wisdom, there's understanding of Tehuti. However; one must become a caring individual as Auset. As she brought back the resurrected life of Ausar as his envious brother Set chopped and dismembered him into fourteen pieces. You see, this is what love is. Love is understanding that your body is the Temple of God. You have got to realize that you must fulfill your own self-fulfilling prophecy instead of Thomas Theorems'. Indeed, socialization is a form of building a nation for the western man. However, the laws of Maat governs the universe. Everything is interrelated. Interrelation is universal and divine love. God's love is universal. By living the laws of Maat, you'll recognize that there must be change in your life by sacrificing things for the sake of love. However, as previously mentioned; do not fool yourselves by allowing the setien world to deceive you with the westernized methods of forgiveness. You see, no one will die for you. Therefore, you must learn the Tree of Life. In this, you know and understand the things of God. You will know and understand the things of the setian world.

You see, mental illness / bipolar is a form of obsessive compulsive disorders of the spirit and soul. In this, the individual becomes obsessively ruined by the following forms; laziness, depression, narcissistic, scapegoat-mania and in denial by withholding true forms of his or her disoriented forms of disabilities. This is of which involves various forms of schizophrenia and anxieties. In this, anxiety and schizophrenia go along with phobias and fears. This also includes excited forms of ideation and enthusiasm and familial boredoms. You see, whenever these kind of individuals become bored various forms of irritation and agitation occurs. This leads to the abuse of illicit drugs by smoking several forms of tobacco daily and inclined to alcohol and drug addiction. This also includes the socialism with various sexual partners. This kind of person has a high pathogen level of sexual excitement by having various sexual encounters leading various sexually transmitted diseases such as; HPV, herpes, cancer and so on. This individual is often unaware of this. This due to the feeling of boredom. This interferes with one's ability of being coherent. Slurred speech occurs often with drowsiness and discomforting forms of disorientation. This has nothing at all to do with symptoms while taking medications. I am speaking of the individual within its own person. On many instances, this is due the birth defects that are with the urethra as well as the uterus and other organs within the womb and fetus. This is due to the varied forms of overindulgence {sex-drugs} of the Maat Tem faculty of the Tree of Life Meditation System. Street drugs play a major role of one anatomy and physiology. They cause a slow death syndrome. Social drugs are known as drugs of socialization. For they disharmonize an individual's spirit.

In obsessive compulsive disorders, these vary in intrusive thought. The word intrude is defined as something that is forced. Something that enters and occupies another space or territory by force. This is like the Japhites and Shemites invading Canaan and Egypt. You get the analogy! Therefore; these are forms of Ideation and delusions of grandeur. In ideation, one has a flight of ideas and never accomplish anything. Yet, the lack of spiritual development, planning, organizational skills and the focusing of details causes mental impairment and damnation. One will become mentally retarded. Retard means slow in the form of movement. Such as; locomotion, motor development, brain development and character of a disabled child. So, these are ancestral disorders as well as embryonic disorders of Bipolar, Schizophrenia, Anxiety and Obsessive Compulsively Disoriented. Those lead to a variety of forms of retardation. Again, mental retardation is an illness that is caused by the condition of delays in two areas. Mental illness is the symptoms of various conditions characterized by impairment of an individual's normal cognitive, emotional or behavioral functioning. Therefore; mental retardation is the dysfunction of an individual's overall growth and development. In addition, the majority of the problem is self-inflicted. Fetal Alcohol Syndrome, Down Syndrome and Hypothyroidism and genetic ailments and illness. This occurs not only during pregnancy. This deals with a disassociation and an imbalanced form of hormones and chromosomes. And so forth and so on. This is due to improper diet. The eating of meats, fast foods etc. This is where one lacks certain vitamins and nutrients and etc.

In many vegetables there are several nutrients that coincide with healing. Here are a few examples; yams, potatoes, carrots and tofu. First of all, yams protect against lung, colon and oral cancers. Yams have vitamin c, iron and helps red bloods cells circulate throughout the body and formation. They also assist in the reduction of constipation of the Irritable Bowel Disorders. Whenever, one is taking various forms of psychotropic and combination therapy, this often leads to other dysfunctions that eventually kills neurons and other bodily chemicals. Those medicines are often coupled with various spinal and nervous system disorders. In addition, potatoes assist in the digestion system that assist in digestion of foods. Potatoes are a great source of potassium. Especially for those with diabetes, lung cancer, cervical ailments, viral infections, spinal disorders, memory loss and autoimmune diseases as well as ulcers / ulcers of the mouth and inflammation. The potatoes source of energy provides the rectum to excrete foods and is good for cancer patients that may also have thyroid problems / cancer-carcinomas and benign tumors. Sarcoma of the uterus {conductivity} / goiters and pyogenic infections etc. Therefore, as yams assist in lung and oral cancers, potatoes assist in decreasing inflammation of the lungs, kidneys, and bladder. Therefore, you bladder will have to be removed. You bladder will eventually have to be removed due to an overindulgence of over the counter medication and other forms of abuses and overindulgences. Carrots are another cancer fighting agent. While tofu is a protein, it aids in the lowering of cholesterol as well as preventing cardiovascular diseases and osteoporosis. Therefore; you must check and correct your diet by living the spiritual and holistic life of which God ordained in your life. I am not making this up. This is done spiritually through meditation and research. Meditation, diet and exercise brings out change in one's life, by growth of the spirit as well as an individual's behavior. Come and grow with me. It's God's intention that you succeed spiritually. In the beginning God created the heavens and earth. We are in the image of God's creation. Therefore, we must live as God intended for us to live. As I write this controversial book you are probable wondering, where do I find my source. You see, God is my provider and I am with him. You see, on page 59 of the Metu Neter Volume 1 by Ra Un Nefer Amen it talks about the sixth division of the spirit. This the motive and power of being through electromagnetic motive forces that are living and nonliving forces. This is to enable things to act upon the physical plane through processes of reproduction as George Washington Crile suggests in his book {A Bipolar Theory of Living Processes}. So what is electrical conductivity? I is as follows; [it is how easily something flows or is moved through something else]. Therefore, here you have in the Pentateuch where it describes spiritual forces and idolatry. Deuteronomy 4:16 You see, the Bible wasn't written for the benefit of the Black race. It is used as a tactic in discrimination and racism. Where is says, 'thou shall not fashion an idol to represent any figure whether it be in the form of anything. In addition, electric conductivity is when something flows through something else. In the In the Ausarian religion this is known as Nekhebet and Uatchet. These are the universal laws that have been established according to the reproduction process of the bipolar theory. In this, the universal that governs the heavens and earth—the entire universe also govern spiritual, times, cycles, and planetary wind directions. As we are created in the image and likeness of God, we too are capable of living as God had intended. Therefore, we must be capable of comprehending the ill-comprehensible. We too have those same powers. However, the western scientist and physicians had knowledge then. Yet, they fail to give recognition to ancient Egypt. The African American has been ostracized during the times of Zeus and

Apollo. Isn't the bible written only in Greek and Hebrew? Then what is the problem! Give credit where credit is due.

We are the periodic elements of atomic and nuclear energy. This was written in my book "Living Organism"! This is how nuclear weapons and warheads were developed by studying races and embryos through various forms of electromagnetic resonance and frequencies. People have the same atomic mass as does the universe and the periodic elements. However, whenever we lack certain nutrients and energies we lose power through overindulgence. We then have diseases such as aids, HIV, cancer, diabetes and psychological problems. And nekhebet-uatchet relates to the electromagnetic conductors of modern science. Something flows or moves through something else. Therefore, your energy and current can be controlled by someone else's current, inertia or spirit. They call this "waymakers" in the church. It is dangerous whenever they say that you have been saved by the spirit or someone else's spirit—study the spirit! This is false individuals role-play forgiveness. They know when to turn it on and turn it off. They say you can become someone else for a period of time. My friend, be mindful and careful of this. For this is quite dangerous. Moreover, in the theory and process of reproduction this cannot be ignored. The sperm and ovum must account for the various identities of which they produce. The characteristics of each individual. Page 148 Crile 1928; which describes a suggested application of the bipolar theory to the processes and transmission acquired through heredity. Therefore, this leads to ancestral disorders, spiritual clans, prison clans by uniform colors, tribes and the rainbow-color spectrum. Therefore, it must explain how the spiritual and physical characteristics of the parents are transmitted to the offspring. Throughout biblical times, tribal warfare manifested as each of them were recognized by race, uniform color as well as gender. This leads to cancers of the sex cells of the ovum within the cervix. We must recognize the fact that bipolar and sarcomas occur often within the reproductive and sex cells. This was explained in my book "Living Organism", To Be A Hew Is Not To Resemble a Hew.

You see, in cancer and bipolar, physicians say that there is a need for anti-neo-plastics for curing and removing cancer cells by preventing them to spread. These drugs are used in chemotherapy to kill sarcomas and carcinogens. All have unpleasant side-effects that causes the individual to become constipated, have diarrhea and become dizzy-nauseated. This may also cause hair loss and suppression. This also causes bone marrow dysfunction. Sickle Cell anemia also occurs. Hebrews 4:12. The soul, body, spirit joints and marrow. Deuteronomy 28:61 Therefore, K-Dur is a medication that assists in the potassium levels of heart function. Certain vegetables can cure these disorders such as potatoes. Potatoes have potassium healing agents within them. This enables the patient to heal slowly. This also decreases the chances of an individual getting diabetes mellitus. Sex cells and reproductive cells can also cause a nursing mother and the unborn infant to have gestational diabetes. This is prior to one getting juvenile diabetes. They develop high glucose levels. This is an ancestral disorder. Where the nursing mother is often unaware of these complications. In addition, lymphomas are blood cancers the affect the circulatory system that causes malignancies. This particular individual then becomes victimized with a variety of anemia related diseases and disorders. The immune system is then affected causing viral infections. Such as aids and other forms of cancers. In this, there are often blood clots that later affect the PNS. Peripheral arteries are destroyed at the limbs. This is relative to diabetes as well as high blood pressure and a low or high levels of cholesterol. This is an extremely high rate for African Americans. African Americans have been affected more than any other race with cancer related deaths. In this, individuals become highly fatigued, have fevers, pain and skin changes. There are also changes in bowel habits. Individuals have white patches around the eyes and or mouth. This is a form of psoriasis. This leads to unusual forms of bleeding and discharge. Individuals have digestive problems—difficulties swallowing, a nagging cough and inflamed arteries. You see, there are several types of cancer. They are colon, lymphoma, leukemia, bladder, breast, cervical, colorectal-rectum, esophageal, laryngeal, lung, oral, stomach, skin, prostate and testicular. This was explained earlier. Are you with me? Moving right along! However, with meditation, a vegetarian diet and exercise you'll notice positive results. The Kamitic-Egyptian-religion allows the African culture to become a more peaceful and healthy generation. This is done by the individual recognizing that he / she is divine, one with God. Nutritionist will not assist you in your endeavors of healing and eating properly. A physician will fail to tell you the underlying source of the problem, which is your mental and physiological illnesses. Such as; stressors coincide with cancers, forms of hypothyroidism, diabetes and anxieties are electromagnetic illnesses and disabilities. They are setiens that are brought out during the reproductive and sexual cell of the ovum and uterus. Therefore, Qi Gong is a form of yoga that allow blood vessels to circulate and function properly. In addition, you must stop the use of the following; fatty foods, fried foods, beefs, sugars, poultry, alcohol, over the counter drugs, red meats, marijuana, caffeine, pork, steroids, heroin, flammable chemicals, crack cocaine and so.

However, you should intake molasses, syrups and bee pollen. This will assist in improving blood sugar levels. Therefore, do not consume peanuts, junk foods, processed foods and or saturated fats. As well as white flours. Calcium, Melatonin and Vitamin D are good sources for reducing cancer and the bone marrow and neoplastic deficiencies. Neoplasm is when the protoplasm in the nucleus of a plant or animal cell surrounds the chromosomes or nucleus. In this, leukemia is easily transferred through sex cells due to immature blood cells. This often leads to cancers of the white blood cells. Metastatic diseases are diseases that have spread from several parts of the human body and has traveled to another location within the body by seeking rest. In Myeloproliferative Neoplasm, the malignant cells worsen. This can cause internal and structural damages to an individual's bones. In this, patients then become victims of various forms of bone cancers. Invasive organs can cause damage to bones. Lumbar puncture, spinal puncture and lumbago are just a few bone disorders. The hemoglobin is yet another form of cancer causing agent. This is when red blood cells are low in this sickle cell gene. These are ancestral disorders. Vertebrae cancer of the bone marrow is caused by tumors of the spine and vertebrae which originated from another part of the body. This is called metastatic cancer. The cancer has spread to the spine. This is from symptoms of arthritis, bursitis and osteoporosis.

As we now understand that metastatic disorders travel throughout the body. Therefore, we must understand that viral infections do the same.

Therefore, in viral hepatitis, germs spread throughout one's anatomy. In this, hepatitis usually creates havoc in other individual's lives through sexual contact. You can say the same for tuberculosis which is also a form of cancer of the liver, lung etc. Therefore, bone hepatitis can develop. In this, spinal hepatitis can occur. Moreover, smoking and alcoholism can also cause TB and various forms of hepatitis. Which can be transferred to another by sneezing, spitting or coughing. These diseases are more common in African American villages, homes and communities. This is due to the lack of understanding by the misleading by the westernized forms of hypocrisy, malnutrition, low self-esteem and poverty.

In addition, multiple drug resistance occurs while taking combination therapy. In combination therapy there are multiple forms of medication given to the patient. This means the patient will have a higher rate of consuming viral infections and mental diseases. These mental diseases include, diabetes, bipolar, schizophrenia, obsessive compulsive disorder, anxiety, alzheimer's, parkinson's disease and dementia. You see, your drug may be your problem. Your drug is your problem.

# THE EUTHYMIC

Normal is used to describe this type of personality. This individual is non-depressed with a reasonably positive mood that is full of energy. "The life of the party". This is known as hyperthermia. Hyperthermia refers to an individual being full of energy with a happy mood. However, this individual is extremely depressed internally. That is hypocrisy. Individuals that have narcissistic disorders will smile in your face and destroy your character and personality while not being in your presence. You see, man's arrogance, selfishness and stubbornness keeps him or her from developing into the person that God has intended. In this, euthymic individuals are within everyone on the face of the earth. You must be saying to yourself, "how can this be". Well I must say that all of man has ups and downs. However, within man is God! God governs man's spirit. That is, if we stop assuming that we are separated from HIM!

In addition, God is love and full of life. Therefore, you must deny self. By denying self-first—you are getting closer and closer to God. God is your true self. Your true self allows you to withstand the tactics of Satan. Satan is your friend and enemy. In addition, Satan will materialize your destiny and all that you are pursuing. This is done with his cunning speech and clever ways of thought. For Satan is talkative, sexual prowess, sensitive, risk taking, repetitious and rarely sleeps. Therefore, I understand that insomnia is a disability. However, there are individuals with these disabilities who are playing the emotions of the weak. Therefore, the weak who aren't labeled with a disability, yet ought to be. It is an emotional rollercoaster. In this world, there are way too many individuals who have a flight of ideas for the lives of others. Yet, they fail to work and re-develop themselves. You see, within the Tree of Life Meditation—there's understanding that in order of one becoming strong—one must become weak.

Weakness is being humble by understanding that God is within every living soul that was created. In Genesis, it says that man became a living soul. If that is the truth, which it is—choose whom you shall serve. Choose what you shall serve carefully—with a clear knowledge and understandings of what is going on. In addition, mental health has gone to hell because it is westernized and excludes God. God is in everything. That is why no one is healing. For reasons of the bigotry of denial of God's Word—The Metu Neter, by Ra Un Nefer Amen I. The message is clear to the point that makes nonsense become reality. Grandeur and delusions are the things that are established by the stubborn western man who enslaved the people of African from the beginning. The bible says that Satan is the father of lies. For today, setiens have and are following in his / her footsteps. Therefore, cognitive impairment and mood swings have seduced the unstable. In this, is your medication healing or harming you. For, it causes memory loss and verbal learning to decrease.

So, hyperthermia temperament is various forms of hypomania within mechanisms of bipolar and schizophrenia. In this, individual often role-play lives of other / one another. By seeking after those with so-called false forms of familial personalities. This is genetics and racism. You see familiar spirits are demons and devils of polytheism. However, Deuteronomy 18:11 is specifically denouncing the people of Canaan and ancient Egypt. For their spiritual ritualistic religions weren't of sorcery, soothsaying and necromancy. Didn't king Saul / Apostle Paul study and those mechanics.

You see, we all have characteristics of the tree of life and the tree of knowledge are within us. The story has been falsely told by western theology, science, religion and medicine for profit. Therefore; the positive euthymic individual has often been characterized a liar, a thief, lazy and hypocritical. In addition, this individual will always be labeled and stigmatized by his her fellow peers, kinship and others. In addition, true familiar spirits are not fortunetelling devices as the bible forbids. Divine oracles give guidance in an individual's walk up the tree of life with God!

Therefore, dysthymia is the externalization form of euthymic. This is where the depression levels are lower in the beginning and later develops as one begins to age. In aging, there's a form of low self-esteem with high levels of anxiety and mood changes. In this, there are several medical procedures that begins to surface. The western civilization calls this psychotherapy. In psychotherapy, there is meditation and music involved. This is where the psychotherapist leads by having the patient visualize his / her person in a more positive state of being. Out of reality. This is also where the client becomes more confused due to the lack of spiritual intervention. This causes man to have a temporary fix. A quick fix does more harm within itself. There is no form of hierarchy and manifestation of the spirit of God. Therefore, you cannot exclude God. Each day is a different personification of the magnification of higher intelligence of the faculties of God's persona.

God's persona is within every living creature on the universe. Therefore healing is the manifestation of God's love for you. In God, there is healing to various forms of depression, cancers, diabetes, bipolar swings and so on. You see, we have to understand the illusions of paradise has been ill-gotten and portrayed by the devil. You know what I am saying! Good. There's several phases of divinity as well as spiritual healing. I spiritual healing, you have the power and authority over strongholds that are enslaving your being. Your body is the Tree of Life. The tree of life is the power of God!

Therefore, unknown depression is considered as euthymic and dysthymic. They, the two coincide with each other. This leads to schizophrenia. Schizophrenia is a mental disorder that is characterized by a breakdown in cognitive and thought processes. This includes negative emotions and the hearing of voices and so on. However, in many this is invoked by the Devil. Your circle of friends are tapping into your head / portions of your brain to manipulate their desired actions for you. For, "we made the son of man". This is written in the bible as well as the Quran.

You see, mental illness is caused by the negative aspects of Sebek. Sebek is the eighth sphere on the Kamitic Tree of Life. The schemer who works as Set / Satan! This is the logical and always syllogism. Which is an extremely argumentative individual. Also, this individual is a slaver of the OCD. The European philosophy was first the African religion. That was brought to the western civilization by Arabs, Jews and Caucasians. They shake your hands and steal all of you possessions. This is Marxism, Capitalism and Satanism. Do you not see this hostility existing daily within your lives?

Axis III DSM mentions that there are mental illness due to a general medical condition. This is called metastasize. Metastasize is a pathological form of the spreading of cancerous activity. Therefore, the mentally ill has faced challenges throughout the history of the world. Diseases and mental disturbances has cause nations and millions of individuals to lose faith in the Will of God! This is by forms of reasoning to the impaired. The impaired, including everyone must remove hypocrisy, bigotry, shame, doubt, fear and want from their lives in order of becoming socially capable of existing in the lion's den called humanity.

Humanity is the quality of being. However, the plan of God has been destroyed by a segregated religious philosophy. In this, we have been overwhelmed by multitudes of syllogism and schisms. A schism in mental health has disharmonized the living God! God's number one plan is for everyone to be healthy. This originated in Ancient Africa, {Egypt}. The bible scholars know this. They have used their intelligence to fool the lowly. This is well explained in the Torah / Pentateuch. In addition, The Quran was written before the Bible. That's another story within itself.

Moving right along! Therefore, abnormal psychology is a much deeper approach to psychological and medicinal techniques and procedures. There have been millions of scholars in the field of psychiatry. However, they have failed to credit those before them. Jesus is not Messiah. There were many prophets who healed before he came into existence. Therefore, the church claims to have healed someone. However, they claim God did the healing. That is two different entities. That is pluralism. A plural is composed of more than one person.

God is monotheistic with a multitude of characteristics that are beyond any form of theories of multiple intelligences. Therefore, individuals with mental disorders are for reasons that are due to a general medical condition. You see; ankylosing spondylitis and cerebralism are brain diseases that affect characteristics of the spine and brain! They are metastasized. In this, there are various effects of mood and personality. This is caused by brain tumors. Brain tumors are caused by infectious diseases such as; Aids, HIV, genetics, environmental toxins and smoking. Therefore, symptoms of a brain tumor range from headaches, leg / feet numbness, seizures, dementia, epilepsy, drug abuse, parkinson's, alzheimer's, head injuries, stroke, static-electromagnetic impulsivities, family history / genetics.

Therefore, this in many cases this is foreseeable negligence by spiritual forces that are racially motivated. Everyone is guilty of this supernatural arrogance by causing a varied form of neurological cancer. In neurological cancer, the lumbar and spine are inflamed with unusual forms of malignancies leading to mental illnesses such as bipolar, schizophrenia, OCD and major depressions as well as anxieties. Anxiety is an inner-state of multiple forms of worry, nervous behavior, pacing back and forth and so on. In this, there is euthymic as well as dysthymic behavior.

This leads to HPV / Aids related lymphoma. This type of cancer is more likely to occur in people who are infected with HPV and or HIV. The National Cancer Institute mentions that the most aids related cancers are Kaposi sarcoma, non Hodgkin's lymphoma and cervical cancer. These are blood diseases and disorders.

Disorders of the Immune system are due to the lack of proper diet, exercise and meditation. This also includes the following; poor medical diagnosis by a physician, psychiatrists and psychotherapist. In addition, this leads to diabetes, arthritis, MS, lupus, poor joints and muscles, fatigue, skin disease and low red blood cell count. Therefore, a negative antibody is the lack of protein by the immune system in response to the presence of antigen.

Antigen is the generator that provokes adaptive immune response. Negative side effects occur leading to cardiovascular disorders. Disorders such as, congestive heart disease and carcino-embryonic tumors. In this, colorectal cancer evolves leading to anemia of the large intestine, rectal bleeding and colon cancer. Resulting from colon tumors. These are medical illnesses that distort the central nervous system while harming other faculties that are within the entire nervous system. You see, there has to be some solution to this form of universal mania bipolar. However, there is no healing by the western man.

# DISEASES /
# SEXUAL DISORDERS

Now that we understand that mental disorders are due to general medical conditions according to Axis III of the DSM. Therefore, mental illnesses are various conditions characterized the impairment of an individual's normal cognitive, emotional or physical functioning. You see, this is genetics and caused by vile chemical warfare which includes various forms of racism. Therefore, through racism in Deuteronomy 28:61 it mentions that the Lord will bring on you every kind of sickness and disaster not recorded in the Book of Law, until you are destroyed. Therefore, the bible wasn't written for the benefit of Black people, minorities and so on.

In addition, this is the divide and conquer rule. In western man's law, we find out that Greece is the main ailment for the world today. In this, we find that history has withheld factual evidence of every individual's salvation. Therefore, each man must work out his or her own salvation with God being the Subjective Realm. You see, scholars have forbidden truth be enslaving generations and cultures for millions of years by their cunning forms of intelligence. However, the godly individual already knows that being informed is not of God. The spirit is of God.

The Quran 18:12-14 informs us on how man was created. Therefore, if this a fact, we must acknowledge that modern health and religion is incapable of healing as the two have said throughout their text. The Ausarian religion is of the knowledge of God. It allows man to choose his / her own course of action. Therefore, they judge themselves by knowing that they are of God. You see, Deuteronomy is a powerful and hateful literary work. It is full of deception and lies told by its writers. In addition, healing will never manifest itself by anyone other than Godly men and women.

Sickness and disease comes from within. From within, we find the nucleus and solution to the healing ways that are only acceptable by God. God heals an mankind is mentally diseased, crippled and disabled by his own actions and lack of wisdom, knowledge and understanding thereof;

Therefore, bodily discharges of a man shall be unclean and cause others to be unclean as well. Leviticus 15:2-8 mentions diseases and plagues that are non-curable. As in Leviticus chapter 21 discusses the rules of cleanliness for the priests. You see, in modern Judaism and Catholicism, There are priest that have preyed upon children, the homosexual and the poor by deceiving them into seeking counsel. By this rule of measure, they have seduced the unstable through rape, torture and false promises of forgiveness.

In this, diseases erupt out of the blue. Out of the blue, unusual cases of metastasizing forms of mania and depression occurs. By this, I must say that the Devil is racist bigot and a cunning liar. Therefore, in sexual disorders, of which, there are many.

1.   Sexual Aversion Disorder

     Is the persistence to avoid sexual contact due to depression, depression combined with anxiety due to distress. Therefore, it can be counted as another physical / mental disorder. Therefore, when presented a sexual opportunity, the person encounters anxiety and or internal anxious attacks. This is also known as euthymic behavior.

This might also include factors such as racial, environmental, disease, and or relationships that are difficult. In addition, this includes family history, incest and or a birth defect.

Therefore, treatment, such as meditation that involves discovering the conflict, difficulties and issues pertaining to life are important in the spiritual development of this particular individual. By finding out the pathogens of your life, you'll begin to understand and accept you disorder and disability by improving you by improving your awareness.

2. Hypoactive sexual desire disorder / Hyperthymic Personality Disorder

   Is Bipolar Disorder and Dysthymic Is The lack of energy or too much energy. This leads to inconsistency in sex drive. Therefore, by taking psychotropics this leads to discharge disorders. This is the sahu and kiabet personality of the Metu Neter Oracle! This also known as HSDD, The hyperactive sexual desire disorder. This can also lead to male and female orgasmic disorders. Therefore, read Leviticus chapters 15 & 21. Do your part!

3. Dyspareunia

   A: This is sexual abuse
   B: Persistent Genital Pain
   C: Substance
   D: Maat Tem
   E: Numbers 5

   You see, you must develop the understanding of working out your own salvation as written in your western Bible of Philippians 2:12. Philipi was too in Greece. Greece was too of the Japhites.

# HOMOSEXUALITY AND SEXUAL ORIENTATION DISTURBANCE

Perversion, Homosexuality and mental slavery are psychological and physiological disabilities. Whereas; mental illnesses are due to general medical disorder. Therefore, Dyspareunia a depression due to incest, rape and or sexual abuse. You see, in physics the law of attraction occurs when individuals or objects are drawn together by a variety of electric forces. Electromagnetic forces tend to often draw or bring things or people together. This is called yoking. Also, in the Kamitic religion, this is called nekhebet / uatchet. This is of the reproductive life cell of inertia that allows energy to be manipulated by force and the will of others to unite in a spiritual connection. These energies can be either positive or negative through karma.

In addition, the reproductive sex cell allows objects to enhance in their development. In this, there are a varied forms of spiritual manifestations that manifests. Flesh and homosexual act aren't what God had intended form mankind. Romans—the first chapter discusses issues of homosexuality, sodomy and beastiality. Read 1 Corinthians 6:9. Also, note The laws of Leviticus 20:13 discusses that if a man has sexual relations with a man as with a woman the two of them shall be put to death. Also, note the story of Sodom and Gomorrah as well as the story of Lot! They all were homosexuals.

You see, this is an ancestral disorder that has dismantled humankind up unto this day and age. We have a problem [Deuteronomy 28:61] with mental disorders. Homosexuality was removed from the American Disability Act of 1973 according to the American Psychological Association and DSM II. Therefore, homosexual genes are of nonsense as many psychologists would say. However, I beg to differ. Genetics and heredity are histological as our current American lawmakers suggest that we approve this vile activity. This is the Second Coming of Sodom and Gomorrah!

The resurrection of Satan and Hell must be excluded from society and the statistical manuals. How can one become cured if he or she has no proper medical and or psychiatrical knowledge as it pertains to this disorder.

You see, homosexuality is of paganism, idolatry and disorder. In this universal disorder, we must overcome this lex Julia form of social hatred by the ending all forms of sin and homosexuality. Homosexuality is a dysfunction of the brain. Its reptilian has been trained to respond in this vile direction due to a lack of meditation and proper diet. Therefore, in this, individuals tend to have both of the following; Sexual Identity Disorder and Gender Identity disorder.

The two are extremely different. You see, in sexual identity, there are situations and circumstances that mental illness rise from. In this, sexual identity is a form of dyspareunia; which is one having too many sexual encounters with various individuals due to one's own forms of depression and idleness. This is where the individual has problems in underlying personal relationships. This eventually becomes gender identity disorder. In gender identity evidence suggests that the individual was born with the presence of white matter and neuron patterns observed in the brains of transsexuals of either sex. This includes longer instances of the androgen receptor gene.

This gene is found in spinal cancers, lumbar puncture, lumbago and neoplasms of leukemia. This occurs in the African American more-so than any other nationality. This is one of the main causes of diabetic obesity, aids, HIV, HPV, tumors, anxiety, stress, bipolar, ADHD, and schizophrenia. There are more factors that include parkinson's, dementia and alzheimer's. In addition, the hemoglobin levels become affected causing sickle cell anemia. Once again, this is an ancestral disorder which causes bone marrow tumors and vertebrae cancer.

Sexual diseases and disorders are the main reason for children being born with disabilities. This is due to drugs taken during pregnancy and lactation. The female may have various sexual partners other than the father / neither of them are aware of the pregnancy. Therefore, there's a continuance of sexual and drug induced activities by both partners. These illness are not only of heredity, they too are of the pathological nature. There is a string of partners—You are / You are not the father syndrome.

Children with disabilities and gender disorders tend to role/play acts of homosexuality and lust by playing house. This happens in the Black community. Communities of poverty. This is where the children wake up to prostitution, gangs, drugs, violence and domestic violence. This is where there's only one parent or guardian in the home. The guardian is either too old, too young, abusive or aggressive in foster parenting skills. These skills eventually lead to destruction.

Sexual and behavior disorders occur when the child then imitates the character and personalities of which he or she has seen by those who are to be watching over them. They gradually become ill-motivated in an educational setting. This is when they are placed in either a foster home or a residential treatment facility. This is when they must remain a victim of various forms of generational curses that has plagued mankind since the European and Arab enslaved the people of ancient Khamit. That is ancient {Egypt}!

With the understanding of Maat, parents understand the principles and nature of God! In this there will be less acts of homosexuality, perversion and birth defects. You see, children become images of their parents. They become images in the likeness of their parents. Therefore, if the parents or one of the parents have an infirmity—/ the child or children will likely have some. This is through the reproductive sex cell act of the union of mating. This lies within everything that breathes life. Therefore, if the parent[s] are overindulging anything, it is likely the offspring will have overindulging behaviors towards something. This becomes fetishisms that are conditioning factors that will eventually hinder the spiritual growth and development of the particular are in question.

Spiritual ritual is healthier than that of psychotherapy. Well, let me get back to my point of disease and sexual disorders. You see disease is an abnormal condition affecting the body of an organism. Therefore, spiritual ritual is the encounter of the spirit in connection with the mantra needed to bring out the internalized conditions of the physical body. Abnormal behaviors and thought patterns are conditions that are controlling the physiological nature of worldly beings and throughout their daily activities. They are spiritual modifications of the Tree of Life in the Ausarian religion.

Spiritual modifications allow individuals to heal in their abnormal behaviors. These behaviors include homosexuality, sexual perversions and overindulging behaviors. You see, the Kamitic practices are practices of which the Old Testament religions, tribes, judges, kings, rulers and priests fail to follow in their arrogance. However, they chose forms of idolatry. Idolatry, such as, rape and homosexuality that causes individuals to be mutilated by the genitals etc.

In this; 2 Kings 17, 2 Kings 19:7 and 2 Kings 24-25 there were several instances where soldiers and individuals commits vile acts of sodomy as they had instances of insecurity. The following tribal nations committed such acts.

1. Assyrians
2. Babylonians
3. Samarians
4. Israelites
5. Jews / Hebrews
6. Moabites
7. Ammonites

Today, this practice began in slavery as Negroes were ostracized by the Greeks and also during both pre-colonial and post-colonial slavery. This then became legal and modernized by 1845 during the Mexican-American War. This also was during the signing of The Emancipation Proclamation [1865] by Isaac Baker Brown. In 1866, Brown described the use of clitoridectomy as a cure for several conditions such as epilepsy, catalepsy, mania, masturbation and hysteria in females.

This has led to a histological form of female genital mutilation. In this, this has become a cultural ritual by ethnic groups in sub-Saharan and Northeast Africa and migrated to Asia and to the Middle East. You see, in this females of all ages are involved in this particular practice. Some are given an anesthesia. Therefore, the health effects depend on the procedure but can include recurrent infections, chronic pain, cysts, the inability to become pregnant and complications during childbirth.

This practice is known as female circumcision. Diseases can occur as a result of this malicious practice. WHO Types I-IV. Therefore, one disease is Dyspareunia. As previously written, there is a relationship of this disorder with victims of rape, sexual abuse and sexual disorders. These individuals tend to have bipolar, schizophrenia, OCD, major depression, hepatitis, HPV, HIV and cancers.

Now, on the other hand. The schizophrenic male has what is called TRAUMATIC AMPUTATION OF THE PENIS. In this, the majority of patients have been known to have gender identity disorders and low self-esteem. This is where they become jealous of their homosexual lovers. The psychiatric patient includes episodes of delusion and grandeur. Hyperthermia also evolves from the pre-symptoms of the individual needing an amputated penis.

This practice is sick and act of lewdness. You see, in western medicine they have excluded God. This is the western way of healing. These individuals have taken away works of divine intervention of the ancient Egyptian culture and practices and materialized it with dogma. As dogmatic knowledge is several principles that tend to believe that something is controvertibly truth.

You see, these are practices similar to those of King Leopold. King Leopold was a king of the Congo. This man committed vile acts of genocide. Did King Leopold and Isaac Baker Brown actually have the pleasure of working along-side one another in this malicious fortitude of socialism? These practices are consistent with those of the gods of Rome and Greece. In turn, this has become modernized slavery. Slavery of which everyone suffers this cruel chastisement of torture.

Therefore, mental illness is of any of various conditions characterized by impairment of an individual's normal cognitive, emotional and or behavioral functioning! You see, the causes of mental illness is shameful and yet disturbing. This is by circumstances that are due to an individual's lack of knowledge as it pertains to his or her mental and or physical deficiency of deficiencies. Therefore, this is like DADT / Don't Ask, Don't Tell!

In addition The DADT policy which came into effect in 1994, while Bill Clinton was commander and chief of The United States of America. This coined the new term "Gay Disease". Therefore, anal intercourse tends to injure rectum tissues. In this, many individuals have diseases such as diabetes, intestinal tract cancers, anal pain, HIV, HPV, weight loss, cramping, diarrhea, fever. Also, frequently loose stools. This is also due the hereditary dysfunctions as hereditary and genetics play key roles in this form of modern Sodom and Gomorrah.

As written previously written in this chapter with regards acts of sexual encounters during biblical wars, these vile acts of lewdness must somehow cease. Society has a whole must be a refuge for counsel for those inappropriate acts of lust and crimes against humanity and God. As I must say, "I am against

homosexuality, perversion and sodomy. These are spiritual conditions that cause more socializational difficulties for each individual in his or her quest for universal independence. Jesus said that it is more tolerable in Sodom and Gomorrah. However, the ancients said it prior to his first breath on earth. In addition, antibiotics such as penicillin is often used as a cure in order to stabilize the pain and disease gonorrhea. You see, aids is also a disease of which vagabonds, male and female prostitutes and those individuals who are homeless usually attain as the seek refuge. This causes arthritis, bone diseases, eye diseases and colitis.

There are various forms of venereal diseases and cancers. They are as follows;

1.  Anal Cancer
2.  Chlamydia trachomatis
3.  Giardia lamblia
4.  HPV
5.  HIV
6.  Gonorrhea
7.  Viral Hepatitis
8.  Syphilis
9.  Herpes simplex virus

Those diseases are disorders that are self-inflicted by each individual due to his / her lust and desirous passions of darkness. The brain has to be constantly redeveloped through meditation-spiritual development. In this, healing begins to take place. This is in opposition of western forms of theology, philosophy and educational medicine. Healing comes from within. From within, we receive healing. In healing, there is growth and development.

Development is health through vitamins, homeopathies, meditation and exercise along with a vegetarian diet. However, individuals have ignored the fact that God dwells within them. Within each of us dwells the periodic table of elements. Therefore, whenever there's an underlying illness, we tend to lack the proper nutrients, energies and chemicals that are necessary for us to live healthy lives. In this, we obtain unwanted viruses from forms of external systems of electromagnetic energies. These energies tend to weaken our levels of oxygen, blood flow and chemicals that are already within us.

Therefore, the following illness become a part of our genetic history and makeup;

1. Aids—HIV—Hepatitis—Diarrhea—HPV

   Selenium
   Lecithin
   Vitamins c, d and e
   Folic Acid
   Rose
   Potassium
   Lycopene

2. THYROID / CANCERS / ANXIETY

   Selenium
   Alfalfa
   Lecithin
   Vitamin D / C
   Potassium
   Folic Acid
   Melatonin
   Ginseng
   Calcium
   L-Tyrosine
   L-Glycine
   DL Phenyalanine

3. MENTAL DISORDERS—MOOD—NEUROLOGICAL—DYSTHYMIA

   L-Tyrosine
   Selenium
   Kava Kava
   Tyrosine
   Phenyalanine
   Tryptophan
   Amino Acids
   Histidine

B Complexes
Vitamin C
Lecithin
Inositol

4.  CARDIOVASCULAR

*See Diabetes and Cancers*
Selenium
Astragalus

You see, those are just a few example. I have taken majority of those vitamins and homeopaths. Therefore, I am aware of the precautions and so on. No one can question me regarding this. Therefore, I am not prescribing any of those to anyone. I am only making you aware of this. This according to my journey of progress in my venture of healing. God knows what is right for everyone. It is his intent to guide my daily achievements and spiritual development. It is also his intent to guide yours as well.

Healing is several processes of submission. Therefore, it is my intent that I'll never become dependent on prescription drugs and die at an early stage of my spiritual development as others have failed to do. In addition, drug dependency and specifiers of tolerance and withdrawel are attributed with a much higher risk for immediate medical problems. As previously mentioned in this book, mental illness is of various conditions characterized by impairment of an individual's normal cognitive, emotional or behavioral functioning. This also leads to a varied form of dissociative disorder. In dissociative disorder, individuals often suffer from lost memory through stress related symptoms. They suddenly become forgetful and eventually become alcoholics by forms of obsessive compulsive disorders and mania. This is due to genetics and heredity.

Therefore, meditation and psychotherapy are necessary due to the patient consuming characteristics of parkinson's disease, dementia, and or alzheimer's. You see in dissociative amnesia, there are signs of multiple personality disorder. However, God too has several characteristics and personalities. And each man has similar characteristics within his or her person and spirit. Therefore, these particular individuals will greatly be fulfilled in the studying of The Tree of Life Meditation System by Ra Un Nefer Amen.

This system is of the Ancient Ausarian religion of (Khamit). Khamit was one of the greatest dynasties of Egypt until it was invaded by Arabs, Jews, Hebrews and European. In this, it has been denounced throughout the Bible. It has been criticized and enslaved by Greece and all of the churches of the western civilization ever since they began recording their history.

You see, this is a phenomenon. The story is true. The story is factual. This is evidence of the malnutritioned western thought and philosophical differences that has enslaved mankind for centuries through arrogance, hypocrisy and shameful forms of hatred and denial.

Denial, by means of deception racism, hatred, idolatry and gay and lesbianism. You see, paganisms are erected due to the fact that individuals have crisis with their identities. In this, there is a linkage within the heredity of all living organisms. All living organisms have been dismantled and shackled by internal forms of mental slavery. This is with regards to their lack of understanding with regards to self. This also includes colonialism which is a post reenactment of human torture and malicious forms of bodily sacrifice. This, therefore, is unnatural sin. Whenever anything is unnatural it brings about disguises of which medical diagnosis become entangled within the chain of darkness.

Therefore, in darkness, individuals become idle in their attitudes, moods and behaviors. This is evident in mental illness as well as other medical deficiencies. Today people with mental disabilities must be committed to change. In change there is spiritual growth and development. In the growth progress the central nervous system is overwhelmed with activity. This activity include karma. Karma is static electromagnetic life forces of Ra. In Ra there is a connection to the Subjective Realm. Within the Subjective Realm we seek to find the root of the problem and circumstances that must be obtained in order of obtaining success.

Success can be obtained spiritually as well as metaphysically. In the spiritual, we find that there is a greater goal of achievement to look forward to. Also, in this, we find that we are in oneness with God. Therefore, you must include God within your every objective. We are the Periodic Elements. We aren't separate identities from God. However, homosexuality within the nationality of mental illness has overshadowed the common illnesses by making them unnatural and ill-curable forms of seduction and lewdness. This keeps us from finding and knowing God.

Lewdness by means shame and doubt along with inconsistent forms of religious thought. This leads to hypocrisy. Hypocrisy is like a sexually driven relationship that is Godless. Christianity is hypocritical. It forgives homosexuality by excluding spiritual development. If there is spiritual development, there is no homosexuality, sexual abuse, lewdness and child abuse that leads to genetical forms of mental disability. As Every form of disability is of the genetical nature. Therefore, in hereditary we find that medical illnesses cause a variety of mental illnesses.

# PSYCHOLIGICAL FACTORS AFFECTING MENTAL ILLNESS AND FORMS OF RACISM

In mental illness there are millions of psychological dysfunctions. These dysfunctions are mainly characterized by religious, spiritual and racial problems. These problems are due to the polytheistic religious philosophy of the Greek Religion. In their belief system, they believed in many gods. Therefore, this becomes racial due to the fact that the Holy Bible was written in Greek and later in Hebrew. This is non-Jewish thought. This is due to the captivity of Egypt and Canaan by the Arabs, Greeks and Europeans. In addition, this also has become mental slavery and many forms of psychological racism. Of course, this is a form of genetics and hereditary. These factors include a variety of patterns of pathological behavior. Therefore, in pathological behavior this includes abnormal thoughts and actions. These actions include abnormal patterns of behavior due to the level of pathological issues. Whereas; this behavior is caused by mental problems and or psychotic symptoms. These problems stem from bad situations and experiences. This can also stem from a variety of forms of hatred through, race culture and religious philosophy.

In religious philosophical differences, the guilty becomes envious of the greater or more promising theological practices of the other. This is by documenting fallacies and creating negative situations about the other. In addition, these could be extremely traumatizing experiences of which and could have visualized in dreams, meditation and so on. Or, they could just simply be portions of delusion and grandeur in a psychological nature. That is why we have The Metu Neter as well as The Diagnostic Statistical Manual. Which is known as the DSM. As the Bible and Morman-Quad denounces minorities and mainly the African American Race. In the Book of Moses (December 30 1830) 7:8 mentions the fact that there was a Blackness that came upon the children of Canaan, that they were to be despised by amongst all people.

This is mentioned in the Quad of the Book of Morman that was written (December 1830) by Joseph Smith during the era of Thomas D. Rice— the founder of Jim Crowism. Therefore, In Moses 7:8 it says, that the Lord shall curse the land and cause a barrenness thereof. This thing shall last forever; and there was a blackness that came upon the children of Canaan, That they were to be despised amongst all people. This therefore is psychopathology. This means that this is of genetic and social causes. These causes are due to hatred and jealousies amongst different races and social classes. In this, we must also note the book of Genesis 9:25-27. This discusses the fact that racism and discrimination due to mental illness and or defect occurred during that particular time.

If this is the case, which it is, we have a very serious problem. The problem is us. We all have forms of discrimination and racism within us. This leads to disoriented mental abilities and so on. In addition, this leads to a variety of generational curses and various mental disorders. Now, extreme racism is a major symptom in many psychotic disorders. Psychotic disorders such as religious and spiritual problems as well as all types of bipolar and schizophrenia. This is also OCD. In this psychopathology is extreme and obsessive through generational curses. This has been a distress since the Greeks, Arabs, Hebrews, Jews and European first observed the religious rites and lifestyle of (Kemet)-Egypt and Canaan.

This is due to arrogance, torture and aggression that racism, bipolar and mental illness exists. In this, psychiatric disorders have grown rapidly within the mainstream of worldly affairs. These affairs have led this modern world into an extreme methodology of psychopathology. The prejudice type includes many environmental and social factors. These factors includes paganism, idolatry and gay rights / of sodomy. This too is hereditary. Racism and hatred are hereditary.

In heredity, substance and medicine abuse can be within this realm of ideological psychosis. Therefore, to be psycho is to be deranged, dangerous and violent. Therefore, a physical disorder can be both psychological and psychosocial disorders according to axis III and axis IV of the Diagnostic Statistic Manual. As mental illness is of a variety of disorders, of one's cognitive, emotional physical capabilities and so on.

However, in racial inequality there have been various slave trades that have enslaved not only the slave—yet also the slaver. In this, for generations, both have become enslaved and addicted to nicotine, opium and alcohol by forms of drug and alcohol related psychosis. In this, this has led to generations of hallucination, idolatry, homosexuality, racism, hatred, prostitution, pimping and forms of sex slavery. You see, in slavery as it relates to the colony of the United States of America, the status of the African usually became hereditary. In hereditary, this is from the reproductive sex cell of the ovum. This is through rape and the process of mating. This is where individuals have been faced with dyspareunia, major depression as skitzo-bipolar. This is mental illness and slavery to the core.

In racism, there has been a long term form of civil disobedience. In civil disobedience there is an opposition of obeying majority of established laws. This is usually done by an occupation of international power. Make note the fact that these are also false form of immigration. Whereas; the first enslaved Africans arrived in now what is the United States as part of San Miguel de Gualdape colony of South Carolina in 1526. Many African tribes were separated by cruel and arrogant explorers. In this, there have been several forms of movements with regards to Triangular Trades. You see, this is where explorers settled in places such as the Caribbean, Jamaica, West Africa, Brazil, South America, the Bahamas, and Florida to capture, enslave and diffuse international cultures. This diffusing manifested by slave, tobacco, rum, gun, weaponry and sugar trade. As there was then the following plantations; tobacco, sugar and rum, there still exists today the same. This too, has become a religious and spiritual problem of hereditaried genocide. Meaning, the inhabitants of those listed nationalities and cultures have lived their lives as the Orisha.

You see, The Orisha's are deities that reflects one's manifestations of God. This is similar to the Ausarian Religion of Kemet. Kemet is the first major religion of Egypt. Therefore, the Ku Klux Klan existed prior to 1865. It occurred as the Catholic Orthodox Bible was written and the Hellenistic Jews were recognized. Therefore, mental, bipolar and racism have erupted from identity, religious and spiritual problems. See, Text Revision DSM IV page 741. Also, according to the magazine "World Psychiatry", human mental health resources in Latin American are very scarce. In this, the estimated figures of 1.6 psychiatrists, 2.7 psychiatric nurses, 2.8 psychologists, and 1.9 social workers per 100,000 are far more below those of Europe or the U.S (1.9). In addition, the majority of Latin American countries devote less than 2% of their budget to mental health.

This therefore, leads to a dismal picture of everyday stressors and a hidden epidemic of domestic violence. Also, in comparing the Orisha's to the Ausarian Religion. The Orisha's do not have all of the tools that the Tree of Life Meditation Systems has. It lacks Geb, Nekhebet, Uatchet, Sheps and Dark Deceased portions as they relate to key life forces of health, receptivity and ancestral factors of guiding one's spiritual awakenings.

In this, as mental health remains a global problem, Africa has a global epidemic of Aids, HIV, Malaria and a variety of forms of diabetes and anxieties. Indeed, there are traditional healers, ritualistic herbalists and so on. However, there are "mad houses" in Africa today that are similar to those during the period of 1850 and 1900. These are call asylums, places of refuge that is offered by the Christian church. You see, we must tap into our individual spiritual source, within ourselves. We must free ourselves from the world's mental and physiological mainstream and ways of self-indulging slavery. Tapping into the power and anointing of God will enable us to be free and at peace within ourselves. This is done through a vegetarian diet, meditation and exercise.

Therefore, the lack thereof is exactly what Satan-Setians enjoy in observing our pain and sufferings. In this, during slavery individuals were fed leftover animal organs and human remains. This is a part of cannibalistic acts of the slaver as well as the native inhabitants of their respective environment. You see, as individuals face poverty today, the following foods are what is eaten in homes; pork chops, ham hocks, chitterlings-intestines, turkey legs and turkey necks. Those are examples of cancer and cardiovascular disease causing carcasses that has been fed to the slave and his / her family for generations.

Those foods cause also depression, anxiety and strong sexual desires and tendencies of overindulgence. Individuals lose their divinity with God. In nature, we are one with God. However, it is the poisons that we are consuming. In consuming this matter, we are further away from healing. Poison is poor diet and appetite. We have been enslaved forever. Ever since the European conquered the African we as a people have struggled. We have also struggled within the holy-spirit. The holy-spirit has enslaved mankind by developing devils, demons and heathens through idolatry, bigotry and hypocrisy. This has been used as forms of mental measurements-manipulating one's mind by taming his or her every form of action.

Every action includes a war on wages for women verses the various women's suffrage acts. This too is racism. This occurred during slavery. Moreover, in ancient Africa (Kemet) there were queen mothers who were political heads and so on. Women were symbols of stability and strength. However, the Japhite, Shemite and Arab often deny social equality towards their mates and women within their society as a whole. You see, in ancient Egypt-Canaan women have also had social equality within their society. The Eastern culture gave value towards the women of their culture and society. Therefore, Auset was prior, through the times of King Soloman. This was similar to Tahpenes. Tahpenes was a queen in Egypt when her sister was given by a Shechem—a king to Hadad the Edomite. It says that Hadad was a storm god of the Semites. This is while God was angry with King Solomon.

You see, the Old Testament is where there were various queen mothers throughout the Bible. This is contrary to where is says women must be silent within the church / 1 Corinthians 14:34. This was written by Apostle Saul / Paul of Tarsus. Therefore, the Greeks, Semites and Caucasian often mistreat their own people by lying. Compulsive lying causes mental disorders and anxieties due to being filled with forms of grandeur and delusional in nature. 1 Kings 11:19-22. Therefore, throughout slavery, European women fought for women's suffrage as well as in The United States of America. This is where The Liberty Party made this a political campaign in 1848. A century prior to Israel becoming liberated. Note, in 1890 NAWSA formed by excluding African American women. This was an Anti-Black women's suffrage movement. Whereas; African American women weren't able to vote until Lynden B. Johnson was president during the 1960's. However, in 1920 Annie Simms was chosen as a delegate to Kentucky's Republican Party. Therefore, this finally became passage in the 19th Amendment under the United States Constitution.

Well, discrimination was written throughout the Bible when it excluded Ausar and Auset. Instead, it mentions Adam and Eve only in the book of Genesis. Also, note the fact that Genesis 9:27-27 denounces the Negroid race and the inhabitants of Canaan. This is slavery, racism and genocide in a nutshell. The biblical scholars had to have known this prior to the bible ever being written. This is a religious and spiritual problem that is mentioned in the Diagnostic Statistic Manual. This too is environmental factors of mental and physical disabilities according to Axis I and II.

In this, there has to be the notion of Axis IV which is that of psychosocial and environmental problems. Therefore, mental illness can also be behavioral and psychological. These symptoms cause individuals to have distress due to loss of freedom. Therefore, behaviors that primarily reflect a conflict between individual(s) and society (ies) / over religious and or political ideologies.

Racial inequality is an extreme form of anxiety disorder. In this, individuals have lost their freedom and voice throughout their lives. Their lives are filled with false hope of delusion and grandeur.

This is within the realm of spiritual darkness. Therefore, this leads to a variety of forms of post-partum depression. In postpartum depression, individuals have become delusional with hallucinations that will cause thoughts of suicidal tendencies. In suicidal tendencies, individuals become extremely maniacal. This incorporates systems and behaviors of high tendencies of enthusiasm and elated misfortunate understandings through syllogistics-preaching—and motivational processes of false doctrines of the western civilization.

These individuals enjoy listening to syllogistic sermons. However they never develop independence and proper understanding of spiritual things. Things such as manifesting the Tree of Life of Canaan and Khamit. For 2 Timothy 1:7 God has not given us the spirit of fear; but of power, and of love, and of a sound mind. You see fear is an anxiety disorder that eventually leads to manic episodes, depression and heart disease. In this, this is contrary to Philipians 2:12 where it says work out your own salvation with fear and trembling. You see Paul's messages were of hypocrisy and lies. He too had knowledge of the ancient wisdom of Egypt and Canaan. Therefore, he wouldn't committed suicide in the Old Testament as Saul.

I think that I have made myself quite clear. For, God uses the foolish things to confound the wise. Therefore, neural and clinical anxieties have been caused by conditional responses. This is known as (CS) conditional stimulus verse the term unconditional stimulus that eventually leads to fear being the "conditioned response". You see, in God, there is no fear. Note, the brain has many faculties that enables one to overcome fear through meditation, proper diet and exercise. Racism doesn't teach spiritual connections of the brain and the relationship with the spiritual behaviors of the the Tree of Life.

Therefore, there is an influx of bipolar in racism and communism. Racism is communism. Communism doesn't only exist in Europe and Asia, it also exist within the churches of America. Chronic health problems are due awe and fear of western medicines. In western medicine, there is no healing. Shameful attitudes between physiological, psychological and supernatural causes of mental illnesses. This is due to bias. Bias is a voltage or current to an active device to produce a desired mode of operation. Therefore, this is supernatural cloning in race, religion, social classes and by political parties. Yes, this is racism and bigotry. You see, the Devil knows the Bible and is capable of speaking in tongues fluently.

If God has not given us the spirit of fear, we understand that we are in the image of God. In addition, we understand where we fit within the affordable health care act and so on. However, fear is often led by anxieties and unawares with regards to one' inner capabilities of unifying within the spirit of God. You see, unity verses segregation and discrimination has been flawed by the politician and theological liar. In this they tell you in 2 Corinthians 6:14 do not be yoked together with unbelievers. You see, this message was from Paul to the Greeks of Eurasia. This too is contrary, as he addressed the Hebrews in Hebrews 10:25 not forsaking the assembling of ourselves together, as the manner of some is; but extorting one another:

Therefore, there are serious problems with this as Paul address the Jews. He addresses them with a symbolic message of love and peace. However, in that particular message, he was speaking as though he was under the laws of Moses that spreads the message of the Torah. You see, this is hypocrisy and racial division. Paul telling one group of people to separate themselves from those who are of lessor spiritual value of prejudice as written in James chapter 2, where is says beware of personal favoritism. This is a religious, racial and spiritual problem that is within the modern DSM IV. In this, this becomes both Avoidant and forms of Dependent Personality Disorders.

The rejections have been flawed with speeches of pleasure and of motivation. Those sermons by Apostle Paul were ignited in order to satisfy his narcissistic ego. He too was a criminal, thief and murderous individual during the Old Testament. In addition, health care and welfare reforms are going up against similar situations today. There will never be peace and unity with all men and women due to their intentional forms of ignorance and arrogances.

Today, individuals throughout the world are facing similar problems as they were during the biblical times. Everyone is selfish and stubborn-set within their own ways of darkness. They are lacking the understanding of love through Maat of the Ausarian Religion. This of which relates to that of Canaan. The two are of which the Bible denounces continuously. This is a willful intent to keep the mentally enslaved, enslaved by captivating their spirits and considering them carnal with indulging personalities of misunderstandings. Those stigmas are then conditioned within the so-called lower class. They then tend to find themselves with numerous medical and mental illnesses. This is a continued pattern of genocidal torture by racism.

What is racism! Individuals are racists towards their own race by the so-called forms of the Holy Spirit. These individuals use scientific methods of racism to justify their wickedness. Their wickedness is like a broken piece of candy that is still inside of its wrapper. Meaning, that they have crushed and weakened the spirit and soul of another by indulging the sahu levels of their divinity. They seduce unstable souls. In this, they attempt to justify their ill-hearted reasons for such vile acts of idolatry that lies within the realm of segregation. They have private meetings and sit-ins to motivate themselves for a short term form of deliverance.

In their short term deliverance, racisms evolve. Racism is actions, practices or beliefs or social or political systems that considers different races to be ranked either inferior of more superior than another. This is due to genetic traits, abilities and or qualities. This leads to social and religious problems within all groups. Therefore, everyone has medical and mental issues that can be identified within the Diagnostic Statistic Manual—DSM.

Indeed, this is a form of xenophobia. Xenophobia is an intense and dislike or fear of people of different cultures, genders, races and nationalities. In this, individuals have anxiety disorders that are difficult to cure due to self-mutilation mechanisms of denial, scheming and methodologies that includes thievery and fraud. This is also known as a schism. A schism is a form of ostracism that includes Jim-Crowism and allegations of war and terrorism. In terrorism, we find genocide, hunger and poverty. This is due to shady political movements that are self-seeking by all means necessary.

If you have studied any form of history, especially the Middle Eastern nations, you'll see that greed has carried it's head unto Africa and the United States of America as well as Eurasia. Throughout the world there has been different kinds of genocide. Individuals have been tortured by lynching, mob beatings, hunger, want and cannibalisms. You see, those are practices of many religions. This goes back to the Pre-Adam times. Times of the Cromagnom. Those people were scavengers and extremely carnal in nature. Those people were warriors only for the sake of survival. They would eat their family members, especially their children. This was prior to the bible.

In this, today, individuals have sacrificed their own children as did the many rulers who are in the bible. Therefore, no one should be sacrificed. This leads to a greater sense of instability and false hope that are within the realm of xenophobia. Therefore, in mental illness, bipolar and racism, there are intentional problems occurring due to the lack of knowledge of God.

You see, it's like a broken record that I must tell you. I tell you that spiritual unification only occurs with understandings of the true Tree of Life. This story began in Khamit-Ancient Egypt and Canaan. You know this. Therefore, the story didn't begin in Ancient Greece, Arabia or Judea.

Throughout modern times, individuals have been recreated by the creation of Human Zoos and People Shows. Therefore, you must figure that out for yourselves by realizing that you are alive today due to many giving their lives for you. This is through God's love for you. You shouldn't be alive today. For, you have suicidal tendencies. The spiritual truth will set you free. You are not you. Therefore, we aren't the same. However, we all are created in the likeness of God. Inside of His image we have been created. Therefore, remove your arrogance. No one person is going to save the world for you. You must work out your own salvation without fear and trembling. For, this leads to an unbalanced spirit.

Kill your pride and arrogance by removing the shield of darkness that has false-guided you up to this very day. God can awaken your spirit. You are a Tree of Life. Therefore, find your niche and let God be the light. He will show you the proper path to choose. This is done through meditation and proper diet. Also, this includes natural organic forms of herbal medicines and supplements.

I have made my message quite clear to you. Are you with me? Good! This is mental illness, bipolar and racism. This is man's form of dictatorship and communism. Have you hear of the I-Ching or Qi-Gong. The I-Ching was rewritten be Carl Jung, a racists. This is therefore scientific racism by usage of lab rats, monkeys and dogs. George Washington Crile too was a bigot and a racist. There have been many involved within this racial form of the peculiar institution of Jim Crowism and Chattel Slavery. Therefore, today we live in a hidden form of this stereotypical chastisement.

In this, there has been a revolutionized form of humor to maintain a universal form of peace. Humor will not, repair the wounds of the individual. Healing will manifest itself whenever the root of the problems are recognized, discussed and recreated within the form of healing through meditation. Prayer only invokes a person to a temporary form of action. However, it doesn't heal the root of the problem. Preaching will not heal. Talking will not heal. Spiritual action is necessary for the receptivity of deliverance of the spirit. Spiritual healing is crucial in this time. However, they are gossiping that the world is ending. They say that this is the "End Time".

Why are they bickering? True revival is a spiritual revival. Therefore, racism, mental illness and bipolar are hidden disguises and illusions of love. Note, just as King Saul used tactics towards a witch as he disguised himself while seeking omens to bring up Samuel, individuals seek power and control of the lower part of your being in order to control your entire being.

In mental illness, we must comprehend the ill-comprehensible. There is no sacrifice during this process. To sacrifice is to give up something that is of value. However, also that thing of value can be something that you had never needed. The Bible mentions that there were many people and things that were sacrificed by ritual. It later mentions that no one or thing shall be sacrificed. In Deuteronomy 12:31 / therefore, a cross is an idol. An idol is usually something carved, made of stone, brass, wood, steel or iron. This is symbolic to the golden calf during the time of Moses. Therefore, a crucifix is of idolatry as too an individual hanging from a tree.

The bible calls this idolatry as well. Deuteronomy 21:23 mental illness and medical illnesses are generational curses. However, the spiritual power and pure understanding and knowledge of God will set you free from masquerades of evil forms of deception.

# MENTAL ILLNESS

M ental Illness is any of various conditions characterized by impairment of an individual's normal cognitive, emotional, or behavioral functioning. This is caused by genetic, biochemical and psychological factors. This also includes social, infection and head trauma. Luke 11:24-26 When an impure comes out of a person, it goes through arid places seeking rest and does not find it. Then it says, "I will return to the house of which I left." When it arrives, it finds the house swept clean and put in order. Then it goes and takes on seven other spirits more wicked then itself. They go and live there. The final position of the person is worse than the first.

Mental illness is actually the main purpose for suicide, crime and murder. In most cases, individuals with mental illness are often unaware they have an illness or are in denial. This leads to irrational behaviors, negative thoughts or emotions. Individuals become arrogant, stubborn and hostile. They begin to scapegoat others with their delusional and grandeur behavior patterns. This inconsistency is sometimes coupled with Bipolar I or Bipolar II.

In Bipolar there are various forms of mania and hypomania that can include high moods of abnormality a much greater form of self-esteem. People then become Cyclothymia-like. They have disturbances of fluctuating phases of mania and depression. These forms include the following; delusions, hallucinations and or other forms of depression and psychotic features.

Psychosis is a loss of contact with reality. Reality is true existence, actual being or existence, as opposed to an imaginary, idealized or false nature.

In psychosis and mania there's a strong sense of empowerment, manipulation and controlling of others. This manipulation occurs as these particular individuals seem to locate weaker companions and seduce them with their perverted thoughts. 2Peter 2:14 and 3:16. With eyes full of adultery, they cannot cease from sinning. They also seduce the unstable and are experts of greed. They are accursed abroad in the diseases of which they are doomed forever. Deuteronomy 28:61 the Lord will bring upon individuals every sickness and disaster that is not written in the book of life.

Individuals attempt to become extremely physically and emotional controlling with loquacious ramblings. This is that they are given to excessive talk and very wordy. In the Khamitic tradition, this is known as Herukhuti and Sebek Tem. This is a very high form of maniacal enthusiasm. Maniacal enthusiasm is Bipolar and Schizophrenia coupled with combination therapy of medications can cause an in-balance in ones SSRI's as well as Dopamine Inhibitors.

These kind of individuals become imitators of others and situations with excessive force of aggression with highly intensified emotional state of being. Luke 11:24-26. They are extreme in their day to day activities. For example; they are lazy and or are excessive compulsive while cleaning, nurturing and lifestyle. And are aggressively passionate during sexual intercourse. They want sex, drugs and alcohol at any cost. They will steal, kill and cause destruction towards others by any means necessary!

Maniacal individuals often refuse the help needed by denial and arrogance! This is Bipolar Mania Mood Disorder-Het Heru Tem

Syndrome. This individual loves to excessively spend and buy unneeded items. This can also be considered "Obsessive Compulsive Disorder." OCD is an anxiety disorder that can be characterized by unwanted recurring thoughts, obsessive behaviors and obsessions. Obsessions are persistent ideas of ideation that are intrusive and troublesome.

These can be dreams, compulsions, uncontrolled desires and major disappointments. They are a constant challenge of one's ego and are in conflict with one's self-image. This is includes cravings and strong sexual urges leading to homosexuality, (ego-dystonic) behavior as well as narcissism and Bulimia eating disorders.

Bulimia eating disorders are episodes of binge eating. Untamed eating conditions and urges satisfy sexual urges of gender disorder.

Mental Illness is a prevalent dysfunction throughout the entire world. Everyone has something of which they're dealing and struggling with in their lives. In this, God is the only answer. God will show all individuals ways in which to allow Him into our daily lives. An individuals' destiny is his key to Gods' divinity. Having wisdom while having and dealing with mental illness, opens the way to understanding gods plan for you. Prayer, meditation and proper diet will allow one to have less stress, tension and anxiety.

In mental illness, there are various kinds of vitamins and herbal medicines that one can take in opposition or as a combination with psychotropic medications. DL-Phenylalanine promotes emotional well-being and memory. It also is a bolster of mood elevating chemicals of the cerebral cortex and cerebellum of the brain. There are others that I can mention. However, I am going to focus on this story, Mental Illness.

# GENETICS AND PATHOGENS

In genetics, there are fertility difficulties that are created by unclean spirits and unwelcomed pathogens. Hereditary Sensory Autonomic Neuropathy Disorder is a severe genetic disorder of the muscles and nerve tissues that causes pain through involuntary movements of the muscles and inner tissues! The fiber nerves (fibrosis) stems from birth through. In crossbreeding genetics, there is the act of mixing different species in order of producing hybrids. This through the channeling of semen through female ovaries in early stages of pregnancy. This can cause various forms of cancer and diseases such as; ADHD, Bipolar, Schizophrenia, and anxiety.

In the Quran 17:31 And not kill your children in the fear of poverty. We provide them and for you, the killing of them is a great sin. As every deed has a consequence. Consequences are cervical cancer, venereal diseases of the HPV and HIV.

In addition, a pathogen is anything that can produce disease. Transmission of pathogens occurs through many different routes, including airborne, direct or indirect contact, sexual contact, through blood, breast milk or other bodily fluids. This also occurs through the fecal-oral route. Hepatitis and E.

Unclean spirits are unseen pathogens that cause unwanted pathogens to occur. In this, Romans 1:20 tells us that the demonic realm can overtake us if we are unaware of certain spiritual systems that have been created by mankind. There's the Kaballah and the Metu Neter. There are various paths one must endure while using those spiritual systems. Those systems can be harmful and yet dangerous if individuals aren't careful. They are somewhat similar in nature. They deal with structures of the brain as well as its functions thereof;

Therefore, diseases occur by direct and or indirect contact with other individuals. This can be from a simple handshake to a peck of a small kiss. Nicotine is airborne. It causes type 2 diabetes as well as heart failure and anxiety. In nicotine, it also causes the following; cancer, depression, erectile dysfunction and death.

This is past on through genetics and heredity. Consequently, unborn babies have been miscarried, aborted and have been known to have birth defects. They have been known to have autism, down syndrome, adhd, schizophrenia, bipolar and cancerous viruses. Those are examples. These diseases have been passed on from generation to generation as well as prostitution. This is to having several sexual partners.

There's a linkage of generational pathogens and generational curses. The same result occurs with uses of alcohol, breast milk and or bodily fluids. Deuteronomy 11:26-28 says idolatry and the occult have committed a great sin against God!

As a generation is within one's family tree, diseases too have generations. Generation is to beget, give birth to something coming into existence. Reproduction and procreation as a form of familial generation. Families may have a history of mental illness, heart disease, HIV, HPV, cancer and or diabetes. In the familial generation, it's the group of people constituting a single step in the line of descent from an ancestor. The same goes for diseases and mental illness.

Mental illness, such as retardation which is a slowness or limitation of intellectual understanding have become a major factor in this world of which we currently live. These individuals do no look like they have an illness due to their environment. In many cases, this is called inclusion. This is when children and adults aren't institutionalized and live in their current normal environmental settings as well as being place within a non-exceptional educational environment.

Aid to the mental health may be a key to the in response to the killings, by Alqaeda on September, 11 2001, The Navy shooting, D.C. Sniper and The Kenya Mall Shooting! All charged showed signs of Schizophrenia and or Post Traumatic Stress Disorder. The Paut Neteru deals with the Tree of Life, spirits, unclean spirits and the lack of knowledge as it pertains to spiritual things.

Spiritual things are invisible. Yet, things that can be brought to life. Romans 1 explains the abuses of the spirit and the uses of idolatry that is behind the scheme of the lower portion of the Tree of Life Meditation System. This is known as the Kiabet level of spheres 7, 8 and 9! These spheres are;

Netzach = Het Heru, the House and the Will of God. This includes strength, victory, beauty and joy.

Hod = Sebek and Submission, Majesty, intelligence, and quick thinking in a positive way.

Yesod = Auset! Humility, Divine nurturing and motherly.

Individuals cannot live this. They have dreams relating the oracle. Yet, they do poorly as it regards to the correct principals pertaining to the universal laws as it relates to proper health and dietary laws of emotions self-discipline.

This leaves us to genealogy of mental illness and disease. A path is a trail, route, course or line of movement. Also, a manner of conduct, thought or procedure. The hearing of voices brings about thoughts of murder, suicide and crime. Or committing activities that might cause harm and danger to yourself and or others. Those are negative aspects of the Tree of Life.

Destructive attitudes and negative emotions lead to a negative line of movement according to the I-Ching and TOLM System. These type of individuals usually find themselves institutionalized mentally. By manipulation, making attempting influence others behavior or actions. A spirit is an influence. This influence should be positive. However, throughout the first chapter of Romans, it's mentioned that people are without excuse. That is narcissism. The Narcissistic personality disorder is characterized by dramatic, emotional behavior which is in the same category as anti-social and borderline personality disorder. That was defined in the DSM-IV-TR.

FEMALE INFERTILITY DISORDERS

1. ENDOCANNABINOID SYSTEM
2. CANNABINOID RECEPTORS AND PROTIEN RECEPTORS DAMAGED
3. MOOD / PAIN SENSATION
4. PNS AND CNS PROBLEMS
5. OSTEOPEROSIS—ARTHRITIS
6. INTESTINAL DISORDERS
7. CARDIOVASCULAR DISORDERS
8. IMMUNOLOGICAL INFERTILITY ANTI-SPERM ANTIBODIES
9. UNHEALTHY EGGS. 1 OUT OF 6 COUPLE FACE INFERTILITY

*OVARIAN HYPERSENSATION SYNDROME*

1. PITUITARY TUMORS, OVARY DYSFUNCTIONS
2. MILK SECRETING TUMORS CAUSED BY PSYCHIATRIC MEDICINES.
3. POOR ESTROGEN RECEPTORS AND DOPAMINE INHIBITORS
4. * BROMOCRIPTINE * BLOCKS RELEASE OF HORMONES
5. HYPERPROLACTINAEMIA—PITUITARY TUMORS ABORTIONS, MISCARRIAGES, BIG BREAST, HEADACHES AND ABDOMINAL PAIN.
6. FATIGUE, ANXIETY AND DEPRESSION

# BIOCHEMICAL
# MENTAL ILLNESS

In biochemical mental illness, there's is the study of biological psychology. In biological psychology, this is called Bio-psychiatry. This is the study of medicine which deals with the biological function of the nervous system in mental disorders.

Serotonin Syndrome is a life-threatening drug reaction that occurs following drug use and disease. This affects the SSRI's and Dopamine inhibitors. The two areas of the brain that's affected are the Amygdala and frontal lobes. This syndrome is a neurotransmitter in multiple states including aggression, sleep, migraine and vomiting.

The Amygdala is the source that allows individuals to process memory in all cases prior to one being diagnosed with one of the following diseases; Parkinson's, Dementia and Alzheimer's. The left amygdala is linked to anxiety, obsessive compulsive disorder, anger and depression. This then causes various psychotic disorders, panic disorder, such as autism, anxiety and bipolar.

Fish Oder Syndrome—TRIMETHYLAMINURIA

ANEB JAH RASTA SENSAS-UTCHA NEFER I

Is a rare metabolic disorder of the urine that is a genetic disorder. Genetic disorders are congenital. Which is existing at birth._____

Simvastatin-Myopathy, Muscle disease of the muscle tissues opposed to nerves

1. Tertiary Hyperparthyroidism
2. Nausea, constipation, vomiting and kidney stones.
3. Hypertension, bradycardia, depression and lacks vitamin D
4. Due to high intakes of meats, cereals and eggs (omnivorous)
5. Hypovitaminosis—stay out of the sun-rickets
6. Causes cancer
7. There's a need of vitamin D-not in foods.

Cymbalta

1. Spinal disorders
2. Diabetes
3. Depression
4. Anxiety

Adderall

1. Autism
2. Bipolar
3. Schizophrenia
4. ADHD
5. Anxiety
6. Drug abusers shouldn't take Adderall

Novolog

1. Insulin
2. Back Pain
3. Heart Disease
4. Weight gain
5. Diabetes

6. Cancer
7. Fibermyalgia
8. Lower lumbar region
9. Anxiety
   Irritability
   Abdominal Pain
   Dementia, Parkinson's Disease and mood changes—
   combination therapy.

Androgel Hormone

Anemia
Anxiety, depression, cancer, sleep apnea, skin rash
Jaundice, breast and penis disorders
Anemias

Oxycoton

1. Cancer
2. Aids
3. Constipation
4. Spinal pain
5. Respiratory problems
6. CNS and PNS problems

Metformin

1. Anti-Diabetic Agent
2. Antidepressant
3. Cancer
4. Alzheimer's, Dementia and Parkinson's

AMERGE—NARATRIPTAN

1. Serotonin Syndrome
2. CNS and PNS disorders
3. High blood pressure, tingling of hands and feet
4. Dry mouth

5. Anxiety, Depression
6. Diabetes and heart disease if you smoke or not

TRAZODONE—OLEPTRO *CANCER*

1. DEPRESSION, SLEEP INITIATION AND MAINTENANCE DISORDERS
2. DEPRESSIVE DISORDERS
3. BURNING ARMS LEGS AND FEET
4. CONSTIPATION, CHANGES IN DIET, MUSCLE PAIN AND DIARRHEA
5. HEADACHES, VOMITTING
6. MEMORY LOSS, PARKINSON'S, DEMENTIA AND ALZHEIMERS
7. SSRI, CNS AND PNS DYSFUNCTION
8. SUICIDAL TENDENCIES
9. IDEATION SOCIALLY
10. UNIPOLAR, BIPOLAR, ANXIETY AND INSOMNIA
11. BE CAREFUL WHEN INTERACTING WITH OTHER PSYCHOTROPICS.

You, see biochemical medications cause deficiencies in other areas of the body, mind, soul and spirit. Mental illness and disease is any condition that impairs the normal functioning of the body of organisms. Disease is also an illness of sickness that is generalized by disorder. Disorders are functions of abnormality and or disturbances. Finally, a medical condition is a broad term that includes all diseases and disorders.

# COGNITIVE DISORDERS

E xceptional education and cognitive intelligence leads to positive learning. However, a Cognitive Disorder is diagnosed when a patient has a syndrome of cognitive impairment that does not meet the criteria of dementia or amnestic disorders. They are often due to a specific medical condition and or pharmacological reaction.

In exceptional education there are several programs that are available to children as well as adults. NAMI the National Alliance for Mental Illness has many chapters throughout The United States of America. NAMI works with adults. While on the other hand, children are able to be mainstreamed by their school's exceptional education department. In this, there are several members of the schools' staff that is involved. The school administrator, guidance counselor, social worker, parent and child seek to initiate a better placement for the child. Whether it is the special education classroom, governmental institution or a regular classroom.

Genetics and ancestry tend to play a major role in cognitive intelligence. The definition of cognitive intelligence is the act of knowing, being intelligent and being comprehensive. However, it is unrecognized in the evaluation process. Disorders are genetic. Mental disabilities are genetic pathogens. Mental illnesses occur due to individuals being emotionally challenged and disturbed.

Syndromes are passed on by heredity as well as touching and invisibility. Individuals with serious medical conditions pass them on through generation. Mental and cognitive disability co-inside with one another. Serious forms of aggression occurs due to individuals being embarrassed by their mental disability. Shame and doubt plays another major role in their delirium, successes and failures.

These kinds of individuals are often seeking praise. This is narcissism, arrogance and grandeur. Early forms of Bipolar and Schizophrenia as well as autism that is coupled with obsessive compulsive disorder. Heru-Tem Maat is a Khametic deity of strength and will used with negative forces of desire and passion. These individuals often need to be restrained and or monitored with modified behavior objectives. Reward systems play a major role on their lives. If you do this, I'll give you that.

Conditioning and shaping techniques are used to manipulate one's behavior. Conditioning is a behavioral process whereby a response becomes more frequent and predictable in a certain environment as a result of reinforcement, with reinforcement being a stimulus and or reward. The response is when human behavior is learned. This Sebek-Tem of the Khamitic tradition which is of Satan.

The only thing that the children get out of this is educated lies. Lies lead to cheating, gambling, stealing, hatred, lust and desires of the flesh. 2Peter 2 in this, many children find themselves in the principal's office institutionalized or dead.

Abraham Maslow's so-called Hierarch of needs state that human motivation is based on people seeking fulfillment and change through personal growth. This leads to the narcissism of the educator as well as the child. This is the Ego of Freud, which means external world. Therefore, 1 Timothy 5:22 says, never hurry to lay hands upon anyone and thereby share another persons sins.

You see, this is common in the exceptional education process as well as everyday life in general. Children are born of a curse as written in 2 Peter second chapter verse 15-20. Children of a curse is a concept from within generational curses and diseases. Luke 11 20-26 it mentions that the demonized was worse than previously after seeking council. Aaron Alexis and Lamar Odom are prime examples of this serious scheme of mental and cognitive deficiency. Their fathers were addicted to some kind of illegal drug.

This Devil is everywhere that is invisible. Individuals have laid hands on others for their own satisfaction of negative healing. This transferring of spirits is a dangerous epidemic. People have ordained this practice for hundreds of years. This goes beyond the theorists and psychologist as well as the psychiatrist. This has been ritualized for thousands of years by ancient generations and spiritual doctrines.

Deities of darkness have overtaken humanity and placed the ill-cognitive in more shameful hard. This has caused learning disabilities to worsen. The elder generation has diseases such as parkinson's and dementia. Yes, their children are of a curse because with their sinful nature they have passed cognitive diseases and disorders unto their young. Currently, this nation has a bevy of murder and crime due to cognitive disorders.

These disorders vary in range. They range from schizo-affective disorder to severe emotional disturbed. In this, individuals are often lost in this shame and confusion. They rebel with no regards for humankind. They are of a curse. We can blame the elder generations for these non-curable birth defects. In this, they lack education and understanding. Their lack of understanding leads to corruption.

This is BPD Borderline personality disorder. Instability and impulsivity which leads to unstable relationships. Hyperthyroidism is Like other mental illnesses, this leads to incarceration, crime and or suicide. These individuals become Black-White thinkers. This is racism, Sebek Tem and discrimination in a negative way. In the Koran it is mentioned that one must discriminate right from wrong. However, in cognitive disabilities individuals lack proper thinking skills and understanding of discernment needed to carry on with day to day activities.

1 Corinthians 14:20 Brothers and sisters stop thinking like children, in regards to evil infants, but in your thinking be adults. This passage tells everyone to focus in internal things. However, with disorders of the brain it is difficult to do much cognitive improving. In this, there are cerebral vascular diseases such as, caratoid stenosis. This disease causes one to lose his or her intellect due to diabetes, smoking, hypertension and obesity. Individuals can also get cancer and have strokes.

The somatosensory cortex / thalamus of the brain is used for coding, storing and discriminating information. This is called perceptual discrimination. It helps the sensory nerves code and recognize the stimuli from each of the five senses. In many cases, individuals who have brain tumors and or aneurysms have lost oxygen to the cerebral. They end up having CNS and or PNS damage resulting from high blood pressure and or heart disease. Individuals with epilepsy end up having seizures that eventually leads to strokes and later alzheimer's and death.

Cerebration deals with several processes of thought, mentation, thinking, thought process and intellectualism. It is good to have a great intellect. However, that only receives worldly and external possessions. The brain is a complicated process of matter. It has millions of functions. However, mankind has lost its liberty through perversions and lust. Mankind has been cursed 2 Peter 2:14.

In psychiatry, the ID-Ego = External. This equates to no positive results. So they give you lithium in order to assist you in your mind reconstructive process. Then you'll end up having much greater forms of mental depressive thoughts. Thoughts of suicide. Thoughts of murder, breaking the law or harming yourself. Finally, you have lost the abilities of recognition.

Discrimination in the Quran means liberty and freedom. 2 Peter 2:19 However, for they promise them liberty, for whom a man is overcome, the same way he is brought back into bondage.

Luke 11 20-26 Mental illness and combination therapy of medications cause individuals to become more disturbed than ever and they have incurable results. Cognitive behavior becomes belligerent behavior and a war against chemical weapons. War against those who provide them. This is the genetics of genocide.

Terrorism, individuals become terrorists because they seek the {Hierarchy of Needs} in a negative way. When God said, "let us make man after our image", it wasn't for the Jihad to be created. I wasn't for gangs to be formed. It wasn't the occult and secret societies to be created as the Quran says in chapter 22:5.

In this, there has been a major recruitment of women and children as young as seven years old in Alqaeda. They involve themselves for revenge after their kin has been murdered. This is for the following reasons; self-actualization, esteem, security and belonging. Many of them, for reasons of psychological, safety, love and freedom from fear.

1. Gaza
2. Iran
3. North Korea
4. Europe
5. South Africa

The fore-mentioned nations have been making chemical weapons and promoted terrorism for the past two centuries. This is a current measure of opposition of the Foreign Policy of the United States of America.

How does this relate to mental illness, biological medicine, biological psychology and behavioral neuroscience? First of all, in this, a condition is a process of behavior modification by which a subject comes to a desired behavior with unrelated stimulus. On the other hand, a behavior is the aggregate or response to an internal or external form of stimuli.

Therefore, any form of biological medicine, psychology and or behavioral neuroscience deals with visual and invisible stimuli. Stimuli in psychological sciences therefore deal with unspiritual thing. It's mainly externalized and the studying of species other that human. Such as rabbits, mice and monkeys. In this, there are toxicologists who are veterinarians who check for poisons. In poisons, there are toxins. In prescribed medications there are toxins that cause negative stimuli to occur in human verses non-human. This is the researchers job. His or her job is to study individuals through neuroscience and behavioral sciences.

Also, in this there is a form of selective breeding. Surah 22:5 and 4:16 shows the chemistry of molecular DNA and RNA has been diluted by individual who are holier than now as well as followers of Satan. In this, millions of individuals have turned away from the holy commandment that was delivered unto them a worshipped the following; Kaballah, I-Ching, Orisha, Metu Neter and other forms of tarotology.

You see, your destiny is you purpose in life that is ordained by God. However, individual lose contact with themselves by living by the means of externalization verses godly. This then cause various forms of mental illness and serious cognitive disorders of the brain to occur. This then becomes pathological, hereditary, pedophilia as well as genetic.

# INFECTION /
# MENTAL ILLNESS

I nfection is the invasion of a host organism's bodily tissue by disease causing organisms, their multiplication, and the reaction of host tissues to these organisms and the toxins they produce. A host organism is an animal and or plant that nourishes and supports a parasite; parasitic diseases are infectious diseases transmitted by a parasite. Parasitic diseases are mainly products of Sub-Saharan Africa, Latin America, throughout Asia and China. Parasitic diseases can affect all living organisms through the skin, anus, vagina, mouth and or sexual contact. It can also be caused by food, water and bug bites. Diabetes, tuberculosis, cancer, cerebrovascular disease, schizophrenia and bipolar depression are parasitic diseases. These diseases are caused by some of the following symptoms; drug additions, cocaine, combination therapy, abdominal pain, weight loss, weight gain, increased appetite-loss of appetite, constipation, diarrhea, bare feet, feces and or hygiene.

Parasitic diseases also affect connective nervous tissue causing connective nervous tissue disease. Connective nervous tissue disease and pathology deals with all nerves. The nervous tissue deals with the CNS, PNS, brain and spinal cord. Delusional parasitosis, mental illness and infectious by great multitudes. In this, individuals become stimuli to their external patterns of thought through irrational thinking and unstableness. Their thought patterns of thought is delusional. Their prowess tend to lead them from house to house. This is in Luke 11:20-26.

Nerves are cordlike bundles of fibers made up of neurons through sensory stimuli and motor impulses that pass between the brain and other parts of the CNS. Nerves form pathways throughout the body. This is known as pathogens. Motor impulses are forms of magnetic resonance that is Nekhebet and Uatchet in the Khametic tradition. These are formed energies that unite life forces. They can be visible as well invisible. In mental illness and infection such as TB, individuals can be infected through the inhalation of air molecules.

In 1 Corinthians 15:16, the sting of death is sin and the power of sin is the law. Infections through injections of drugs such crack cocaine, interferon, novolog, and marijuana leads to Deuteronomy 28:61. You'll have incurable diseases that aren't written in the bible. Such as Herpes, Diabetes, various forms of Depression, HPV, HIV and cancer of the brain and so on.

Infection is caused by everything that exists in this world. Nothing is safe. We must be careful and mindful of uncleanness. Leviticus 5:1-3 If he touches the uncleanness of the man, whatsoever uncleanness it be that a man shall be defiled withal; and it be hid from him; when he know of it he shall be guilty. 1Timothy 5:22 do not be hasty in laying hands on anyone and do not share sins with anyone. Keep yourself pure.

What is pure? Pure is unmixed with any other matter. Pure is spotless and free from dirt, dust and or taint. James 1:23! Therefore, infection and mental illness has been going on since the beginning of creation. This is due to the fact of idolatry and animal sacrifice. Individuals have used tarot decks in order to help enhance their abilities of becoming one with Baal instead of the Creator of the universe. These individuals have found ways of becoming one with an idol. Such as a beast, creature, the stars, the sun and moon.

They have taken on several spirits while others have entered them. These spirits travel as pathogens into other individuals as they are forms of stimuli that's causes negative conditions and behaviors to manifest. You'll have diseases of the brain through destinational pathogens. These destinations of diseases can be environmental and biophysical. The physical and biological factors along with their chemical interactions that affect an organism is like a parasitical disorder. These people have no regards for humanity.

Psychiatry plays a major role in the DNA of all living organisms that are in the world of modernity. The modernization of Sihu is one who has been hypnotized and a cursed child as a form of ritualized enchantment. This causes biochemical anxiety, negative changes in mood and a hostile state of emotions. This is a form of disoriented stimuli that will eventually lead to abnormal behaviors. Behaviors that have been begotten from the devil. Some have said that man is from a seed and or a soil. They also have said that we have created man form a germ and we will have control over whatever undertaking and life processes that he goes through.

In infection and mental illness, the entire world is involved. However, millions are unaware of this form of psychosis. The Quran says, "We created man from dust"! Sounds like the devil has connected with humankind in order to fulfill his willful mission of polluting the universe. This is by all means of disorder and disease. Disease and disorder has caused the world to be a form of delusion and grandeur. Its people are arrogant and mockery. God cannot be deceived or mocked. However, individuals have called deities and brought about omens in order to fulfill their fleshy desires. Desires of lustful sin and greed has delivered them into cunning exhibitions of idolatry.

In this writing, it has been extremely difficult for me. I must say that God is with me in this un-hasty endeavor. It's got to be to the point and factual. This is due to the high volume of crime, violence, pedophilia, homosexuality, perversion, psychosis and infection. Yes, indeed, this world is racist as it comes to healthcare and mental health. We must put an end the desirable pranks of Satan's Government by cleaning up our own lives. This is by not being evil speaking faultfinders of others. We have lots of work to do in order of fulfilling God's holy commandments. In the field of health and medicine, we need change. Change occurs only all sides put away their hidden agendas in order to find positive solutions instead of recreating ways of biophysical and biochemical forms of negation. This negation will only lead us to moral and a much greater form of physiological and self-destruction.

Physiological is the study of all living organisms. This also includes how cells, organs and organisms carry out the chemical or physical function that exists in a living system. Insulin for example helps reproduce cells that have been lost in Type 1 and 2 Diabetes. Penicillin is also used in diabetes, celiac disease and depression.

Celiac disease is a wild condition that damages the lining of the intestine and causes prostate cancer, HIV and HPV. This is also from eating too many fibers that cause a high form of carbs to produce fat around the lining of the abdomen. This causes obesity, bloating, lactose intolerance and diarrhea. Sickle-cell disease is another blood disorder that is characterized by infected red blood cells. Individuals have infected hemoglobin genes. This too is a disease of heredity. In this, it can be an oncoming disease of psychiatric, HPV, HIV and TB. Hyperthyroidism is also caused by this physiological disorder.

Also, individuals with the listed diseases are given INTERFERON-AFINITOR! Some individuals have been known to have comas, heart disease, diabetes and anxiety. In this, Leprosy and Tuberculosis are formed by bacteria mycobacterium tuberculosis. Leprosy is another form of The Human papillomavirus. This can be genetics that is caused by damaged peripheral nerves and mucosa of granulomas. This is when the immune system attempts to remove substances / particles that it perceives as unable to eliminate.

Therefore, these illnesses are incurable and dangerous especially if contracted by any kind of contact. Tissues and organs are harmed by association of unclean cells, the lack hygiene and the inconsideration for the health of others. This is the selfishness of humankind. Now, in Third World countries this is worse than in the United States of

America. Bee stings cause infectious diseases such as Aids, HIV, Malaria and others. Medicines for those illnesses make matters far more than before.

In this, misdiagnosis plays a major role in the future lives of patients. Misdiagnosis is an inaccurate assessment of the condition of a patient. Harm is then inflicted on the patient forevermore. This is from prenatal to elder. These are from the connective tissues, sutures, nerve cells, nerves, bones and the brain. This also includes arteries and organs as well as membranes.

Therefore, it is useful to seek guidance for other possible illnesses that have been misdiagnosed and what other alternative measures must be considered relating to the diagnosis. Your physician may have already been aware of the alternatives. This causes pain, distraction in your emotions, anxiety and other forms of depressive thoughts. This pain can also cause brain damage such as tumers, concussions, tremors, chronic brain dysfunction and traumatic brain disorders.

In chronic brain dysfunction, it can be from prenatal birth defects and lactose disorders. The leading cause for infant mortality during the first year include the ingestion of drugs and alcohol. Birth defects are major physical anomaly. This the destruction of the babies looks. Its physiological development. Many babies are born with genetic disorders and diseases as well as hereditary disorders.

The pituitary and embryo may have diseases due to miscarriages and infectious diseases. Infertility is the inability to conceive a child due to poor ovulation disease of the DNA. Ovarian cancer occurs from smoking. In this, the DNA damages the male sperm caused by oxidative DNA damages, smoking and xenobiotic processes of the fallopian tubes. Drugs, diabetes, thyroid disorder, adrenal disease, hyperprolactinemia and chemotherapy are results of embryo disease, birth defects and miscarriage.

Also, the uterus and urethra is cancer forming from STD's. This is HPV in male and female from which is from the following; genetic, hereditary and the Paut Neteru. This is idolatry, the worshipping of familial spirits and animal sacrificing religions. Also, from omnivorous lifestyles. One can also have pelvic inflammatory disease due to advanced paternal and or maternal age.

In this, the autonomic nervous system which is located in the ganglia of the PNS has deficiencies. This system causes the motor nucleus of the vagus nerve to become dysfunctional within the sympathetic nervous system. These nerves respond to the arousal energy that is generated by motor and developed stimuli. Therefore, infection, mental illness, lactation and pregnancy disorders often cause children to have special needs, such as learning disabilities and or emotional and psychiatric disorders.

Now, salivary gland infections are prevalent and are from the diabetic maternal and or paternal gene. This can be very harmful and life-threatening. Which is from the arousal nerves which cause the sexual organs to become aroused. Aroused by the means of sin, oral sex and fornication. Also, the motor developmental stages of the reptilian / hippocampus cause the pleasure of arousal to manifest. In this, deity, there are major disappointments that often occur. This leads to stressors that hot and moist energy to occur. Like animals, this individual must be tamed / sterilized by injection.

Het Heru is a combined source of hot and moist—hot and dry energy. Energy from the sun and planet Venus. When combined it should actually be strong, full of joyful and sweet energy with God being the head and not the tail of all current worldly activities. Deuteronomy 28:13 the Lord will make you the head and not the tail. If you pay full attention to the commands of the Lord your God and correctly follow them. You will always be at the top and never at the bottom.

Therefore, as children enter the world, they are blind to its activities. In this, they have unstable souls and are vulnerable to the affliction of Satan. During birth, they are given several test for motor development and reflexology. These are given in order to find out what capabilities or disabilities an infant might have in later stages of development. However, contrary to the eastern philosophy, destiny readings are given in order to find out what kind of child one will have as well as its name and destiny.

This is racism in health and medicine according to the western civilization. In this, in westerners have no purpose in life as well a lack thereof self-sufficiency and self-control. So, humanist have developed racially bias forms of behavior modification skills and techniques in order to maintain control over certain cultures, societies and races. Which leads to a greater form of infection and mental illness in the following areas;

1. Motivated Behavior—sexual arousal of the autonomic nervous system.
2. Sensation and Perception
3. Motor Development—lack of self-control.
4. Learning and memory
5. Sleeping / Biological Rhythm of Emotions
6. Biochemical, Behavioral and Neuroscience Mechanisms.

This also includes, PTSD as diseases and disorders are misdiagnosed. Also, the following; Celiac disorders, ADHD, Irritable Bowel Movement, Lime Disease and Alzheimer's. Those are just a few examples. In this, ovarian disorders and infertility occurs.

# MENTAL ILLNESS AND BEHAVIORAL FUNCTIONING

In mental illness and behavioral functioning there are a great deal of manifested mechanisms that must occur. In this process, there are several steps and procedures that must also manifest themselves. First of all, one must be non-hasty and wait on God for deliverance. Secondly, one must be patient and live Gods' Word. As God healed millions of sick individuals throughout the Bible, individuals can be stabilized with the aid of a good physician and or psychiatrist. You see, there are various situations that bring about mental illness and behavioral disorders. This does not only occur within the educational process. However, it also occurs within the environment of which an individual is nurtured and maintained. The maintenance of these deficiencies must be observed daily. Record keeping strategies must be within a reasonable form of evaluation.

In emotional and behavior disorders (EBD) this is a broad category that is commonly used in all living settings. Racism is organized and controversial. This leads to the occurrence of various forms of emotional disturbances and hostilities throughout an environment. Factors can include biophysical, psychodynamic, cognitive and behavioral. This can also be ecological. In this, an ecological niche is the way of life of a certain species live throughput a certain environment. This is better known as adaptation. In adaptation, individuals often have difficulties adapting to certain environments due to their previous environments.

Previous environments can cause one to have post-traumatic stress disorders and misdiagnosed symptoms of cognitive impairment. In cognitive impairment, learning is obstructed by stimuli and neutral waves of magnetic life-forces of the ecosystem. There are several kinds of ecosystem. Yes, universal laws come into play with interaction through intermingling.

You see, the Bible tells individuals not to intermingle. The Quran tell us to discriminate right from wrong. The Metu Neter Oracle and I-Ching tells us that all things are interrelated. Now, the two are of non-western cultures of spirituality. Therefore, idolatry comes in the picture. This is where social and economical differences are involved. This is also a determining factor of an individual's future. What is as stake in ones' divinity. Divinity identifies the destiny of an individual. However, certain people have taken for granted what God has already provided them. They become scoffers, thieves and mockers of the Creator. This is by all means of selfishness and stubbornness.

This leads to a greater form of anxiety and mental-emotional disabilities. Organic and environmental influences occur in this wide range of disabilities by uses of drugs, alcohol and other related forms of interacting chemicals. Chemical change occurs when a substance combines with another to form a new substance. This is also called combination therapy. Combination therapy is the method of treating disease through simultaneous uses of a variety of drugs in order to eliminating or control biochemical causes of the disease itself.

The use of multiple agents to treat a certain medical condition such as; cancer, diabetes, thyroid disorders and mental disorder. This includes mood disorders such as; manic, bipolar, hypomanic, depression and persistent depressive disorder. These disorders produce negative results in one's cognitive functioning. Double and Triple depression occurs. Yet, children and individuals living in poor environments are unaware of these factors. These factors can facilitate throughout the life of the individual. This is pathophysiological and the pituitary is harmed due to the uses of various medications. Low levels of neurotransmitter serotonin leads to inbalances that result in mental health symptoms. They are;

1. Adrenal dysfunction
2. Blood sugar imbalance
3. Food and chemical (medicine) allergy
4. Hormone imbalance—poor estrogen levels
5. Nutrition deficiency
6. Serotonin/Dopamine/Noradrenalin imbalance
7. Stimulant Drug Intoxication—ANS Autonomic Nervous System—Peripheral Nervous System
8. Under / Overactive Thyroid

Behavior is a range of actions and mannerisms made by organisms and systems. Ephesians 6:12 for our struggle is not against flesh and blood but against rulers, against authorities and against powers of this dark world and against the spiritual forces of evil in the heavenly realms. Therefore, leaders have created strategies and techniques of strategic planning and procedural philosophies and methodologies in order of maintaining their wealth in their greed. Their greed has caused America to become dis-equalized nation. This is due to the lack of a stabilization of welfare for modern humanity. In this, we have to teach ourselves how to read and write soundly while in the embryo. We must have a nourished diet regardless of our source of income.

The education system and mental institutions cannot cure the behavior, physiological and economical wounds of this modernized form of mental slavery. Mental slavery has caused individuals to have abortions and murder the innocent. You see, we must first become unified with others to have a positive supporting cast. This supporting cast will veto the wicked and rulers of darkness. Those who are in high places must reserve their greed by understanding the needs of others.

This is giving and sharing. Yes, indeed, there must be a solution. That solution is God. God and love is unity. No one can lose without having either. Mental behaviors will be accessible in understanding through recognition of certain spirits that are involved. In studying the spirits, it is easily recognizable to the eye of the beholder.

The behavior is less conditioned by the autonomic nervous system and highly motivated to attain achievement and self-esteem! Some teens have behaviors that similar to and worse than adults. However, in ADHD these individuals are unable to finish what they have started. They are easily seduced to given in to gratification. That is narcissistic disorders with maniacal forms of bipolar. This is the empowerment of spirits Luke 11:20-26 and the seven laws of the Mental Health Act of the 29 U.S.C.A. Parity in mental health and substance use disorder benefits.

There are several forms of behavior disorders;

1. Compulsive eating disorders
2. Borderline personality disorder
3. Oppositional defiant disorder
4. ADD
5. ADHD
6. Intermittent explosive disorder, impulsivity, gambling and so on (IED)
7. Reactive attachment disorder
8. Social anxiety disorder
9. Passive aggressive disorder

*Cognitive disorders*

In this, Surah 22:5 says that we created you from dust, then from a small life germ, then from a clot of flesh, then from a lump of flesh, complete in make and incomplete, that we may make clear to you. And we cause what we please to remain in the womb till an appointed time. We bring you forth as babies, then that you may attain your maturity.

You see, this is the Devil and the Bible that has been deceiving the Holy Spirit. Sarin Gas and chemical weapons are used in the taming of neurotransmission disorders as well as medications of psychiatry and diabetes. The Paul Langerhans Disease occurred in berlin in 1869.

This is when he found that his pancreatic cells were producing insulin to fight the disease diabetes. However, he died of diabetes and cancer in 1888.

Moving right along, there are several famous psychologist who have played a major role in this organized form of genocide. They are as follows;

1. Wilhelm Wundt—Experimental Psychology
2. Gestalt—Theory of the Mind and Brain
3. Alfred Binet—Practical Intelligent Test
4. Mary Ainsworth—The Attachment Theory
5. Theologians

In this genocide, we have Adolph Hitler, a Jew, executed millions of Jews. On the other hand, Bashar al-Assads regime of the Baath Party has used sarin to murder thousands of Syrians. This has lead to the Iranian nuke program and its continuance of the promoting of its regime of terrorism against Israel. This behavior is belligerent. They are radical. They are a group of war raging imbeciles. These are radicles. They plants growing to emerge as a form of germination. The seed of the seed syndrome.

Genesis 1:11 is of cognitive and pathological behavioral disorders through ancestry. Luke 11:47 "woe to you, because your build tombs for the prophets, and it was your ancestors who killed them". Yes, outward, these were experts in the law. But inwardly they rejected the message and the Messiah! This is the message that has been written for years and many individuals have forbidden the truth and turned it into lies and worshipped four-footed beast and creatures instead of the Creator. Romans 1 individuals are disobedient to parents. For they knew God. However, they deny God as their foolish hearts were darkened.

Darkened with arrogance, pride and malice with wild forms of hippocracy. Lies are mental and emotional behaviors. They are false statements made by a person who knows that it isn't the truth. Bullshit is often used to make the audience believe that one knows more about the topic by feigning total certainty and making probable predictions. These are false prophets. They are wolves in sheep clothing. Jude chapter one mentions the sin and doom of ungodly people.

You see, ostracism, which was under the Athenian democracy began in Greece. In this, any citizens can be exiled from the city-state of Athens for ten years. Thousands of years later, there was the Jim Crow era. The Jim Crow era lasted throughout the twentieth century and still exists today. There were segregation laws throughout decades of the 1950's and today this still exists spiritually.

No one can have civil rights if he or she is challenged by forms of psychosis and hypnosis. Individuals are devils seeking to snare and seduce the mentally challenged and unstable. We have lost something that we've never had. That is our mind. Through psychologist of old as well as the modern day psychiatrist. We've have never had our right mind. We as a people have got to understand that we're not in this game as a loser to unrighteousness. We have forgotten our sense of freedom. That freedom is with God. We've lost our passion of true love. God's love. The moral understanding the brought creation as a unification.

No one should be denied freedom by meager forms of philosophy and psychiatry. Everyone has the right not to riot. Rioting by Tea Party members is absurd. This causes tension. Mental tension and anxiety that hide God's presence from amongst us. Brain games by those that provide us with forms of experimental medicine and psychiatry.

Mental behaviors become negative when neurons and nerves are disturbed. Therefore, beware of personal favoritism. Personal favoritism leads to spiritual wickedness, racial discrimination, infection and mental illness. Let me explain! This kind of thing comes from within experimental psychiatry. In experimental psychiatry animals are given several cognitive and behavioral tests. In this, the animal is given certain kinds of stimulation. In this, the animal is given a reward system. A reward system is critically involved in mediating the effects of positive or negative reinforcement.

Now, in the spiritual world, man has made several substitutions. This is by replacing one thing with another. They are called way-makers. Way-makers are other forms of items used to replace the original being. This can be a person or an object, such as a doll, picture and or sex toy.

In addition, this leads to racial discrimination and mental illness due to things and people being replaced for different objects. These objects only are used for particular time for specific purposes. Therefore, they aren't used consistently. Discrimination then involves the overbearing empowerment of self-centered, lustful and greediness. In this form of negative discrimination, the PNS, CNS and ANS are distracted and harmed. Individuals become mentally disoriented and social unstable.

Doctors too are negligent. They are aware of the complete findings regarding a persons' health and personal welfare. Yet, they desire to continue to poison their lost clients with chemical weapons that are in the form of a pill. Majority of these doctors are from overseas. They practice not according to their culture. However, they practice according to their pockets and how much wealth he or she can gain from this session.

American Greed is a motha-fucka. You see, individuals must first gain knowledge of their illness. Patients must make their physicians aware of this and report them if there is no balanced compromise. Finally, Healthcare is the greatest and wealthiest field in the world. We need honest individuals to assist us in the achievement in conquering infection and mental illness. James 2 Do not disregard an individual because he or she is poor.

# THE HEAD AND MENTAL ILLNESS

The head is the upper part of the body in humans joined to the trunk, by the neck, containing the brain, eyes, ears, nose and mouth. The head is also considered as the master of the intellect, thought, memory and understanding. Also, the center of emotional control of the mind.

Now, during birth, head injuries occur as a result of uninformed forms of malpractice. In this, Caput Succedaneum occurs. Caput Succedaneum is caused by too much or too little amniotic fluids that are within the uterus. Pressure within the scalp of the newborn also causes this disorder. It is also brought on by pressure from the vagina and or uterine wall during the head first vertex delivery. This can also be caused during c sections. This can cause cancer and diabetes of a newborn.

This is due to a prolonged and difficult delivery. This is especially true after the membranes have been ruptured because the amniotic sac is no longer providing as a proactive and protective cushion for the baby's head. Also, in this, the vacuum extractions can also enhance the chances of a Caput Succedaneum of which an ultrasound can detect prior to labor. This is associated with premature raptures of the membranes or inconsistency flow of amniotic fluids. Finally, the longer the amniotic fluids are healthy and consistent the less likely the Caput Succedaneum is diagnosed.

Surah 22:5 Preeclampsia occurs whenever women have had difficulties during previously pregnancies. This can also be caused by the following; family history, race-afro American, hypertension, diabetes, lupus, renal artery disease, stress and so on. This often leads to a baby born with chromosomal abnormalities and Hydatidiform mole. This is a result from the overproduction of tissues that are to develop in the placenta. This can be a result of one having no fetus and the placenta is abnormal or partial.

This leads to the following:

1. Hyperthyroidism-Anxiety
2. Strokes
3. Depression
4. Menopause
5. Trembles
6. Tremors
7. Inconsistency in weight
8. Cancers /
9. Hot-Cold sweats
10. Vaginal Bleeding / Bloody Urine
11. Mood swings-Bipolar-pre and post (hysterectomy)

Also, Torch Complex is an infection passed on from a pregnant woman to her fetus! These infections can also be STD's. In this, Subgaleal and epidural hemorrhages can occur and cause the following; neonatal herpes complex, HPV, Diabetes and HIV. Diseases can occur throughout the body. However, mainly within any open area such as; eyes, finger nails, mouth and ears. Also, within the rectum and or chromosomal area. These are caused by blood clots within the head and skull. Blood must then be vacuumed while within the head and skull during birth. This also cause problems within the CNS and PNS. All races are affected by this form of prenatal genocide.

This also depends on the environmental establishment and condition of a particular individuals residence of his or her subarachnoid. This is the space between the arachnoid and pia mater. The pia mater is near the brain and spine which causes cerebral spinal disorders. Then then affects the sensory development of an individual who has had lower and upper lumbar injuries as well as spinal and head injuries.

Meningitis is another cause of these carcinomas. This is due to cranial nerve damage. This is called neurofibromatosis. Indeed, this is a malignant brain tumor. Also, the newborn may have jaundice, anemia and or hypertension. In this, the newborns lack vitamin K for several reasons. Vitamin K passes through the placenta poorly and the levels of breast milk and the gut flora has not yet been developed. Therefore, vitamin K is produced by bacteria in the intestines. This causes the following;

1. Mental illness
2. OBD obsessive compulsive disorder
3. ADHA Attention Deficit/Hyperactivity disorder
4. Skin disorders
5. Anxiety
6. Respiratory Tract infections
7. Eczema—Atopic Dermatitis
8. Inconsistent stool
9. Genital disorders—Genitourinary system disorders
10. Urinary disorders
11. Urethra disorders
12. Vaginal disorders
13. Amenorrhea
14. Female genital malformation
15. Pregnancy loss
16. Double vagina

Through alcoholic jaundice, this is hepatitis (inflammation of the liver) through an excessive intake of alcohol. Hepatotosis is downward displacement of the liver. This is liver become serpent-like in its form. In this, jaundice occurs. Jaundice is yellow in color within the skin and or mucus membranes as well as the eyes. Also bilirubin occurs. Red blood cells begin to die. This often leads to various forms of anemic. Sickles are then formed as individuals began having epileptic seizures. This can lead to stroke, tumors and chronic brain dysfunction. In this, the bilirubin accumulates the number of producing cells.

Various autoimmune diseases can occur. They range from all forms of hepatitis, cancer, and pathogens due to the lack of energy within the hemoglobin. There are other illnesses that can occur within this important letter. Cholestasis, which is a blockage of oxygen to the liver. Therefore, a common cause of jaundice is a drug induced cholestasis, the number of medications, mix drugs and combination therapy. Once again, from birth to elder individuals have several kinds of liver cancer. Often, individuals have every form of hepatitis.

These diseases cause vomiting, seizures, brain hemorrhaging and brain damage and so forth and so on. Therefore, when a newborn is in the womb is has an infected placenta. The placenta removes bilirubin from the newborn's liver. The placenta is the organ during pregnancy that feeds the newborn. However, the placenta becomes damaged through jaundice. In this, breastfeeding can produce several kinds of jaundice. This occurs especially when a newborn is often nursed. This is also noticed resulting from toxins in the breast milk and of over the counter milks. Breast milk jaundice is different form breast feeding jaundice.

Blood type mix-match occurs from the mother and the baby leads to cephalohematoma. Cephalohematoma is caused by a very difficult delivery. High levels of red blood cells are common due to a great lack of certain proteins. Therefore, certain medication cause congenial infections. These infections are Cystic fibrosis, Syphilis, Diabetes, Rubella and so on. Genetic disorders as well as heritage disorders often occur in myalgia during pregnancy.

# MYALGIA AND PREGNANCY

C ommon causes of myalgia in pregnancy are overstretching of a muscle and viral infections. This is due to Diffused myalgia, jaundice and walking symptoms in pregnancy. These individuals can get negative symptoms from walking while pregnant. They can result in the following; pelvic disorders, increased lumbar lordosis, lower back stenosis, uterus discomfort, constipation, hormonal changes causing laxity in joints, depression, anxiety and chronic fatigue syndrome.

In this, the pregnant woman can get a ruptured and inflamed gallbladder which is cancerous. The pregnant woman can also get acute pancreatitis. Acute pancreatitis is an inflammation of the pancreas. It can have severe complications despite treatment. The causes of pancreatitis are carcinoma-cancers, alcohol, ulcers, malnutrition, poor diet, drugs and nicotine.

Also, viral hepatitis (inflamed liver) and infectious jaundice are combined illnesses due to feces and the licking of the urine of mice by house cats or dogs. Leptospirosis is found in blood and the cerebrospinal fluid causing hepatitis in pregnant women and they transfer the disease unto their newborn.

All living organism can be plagued by infectious diseases. In this, the genome prosess and the history can be extremely vaccinationable. In this, from overstretching the uterus the unborn can have complications of the following; diabetes, cancer, hyperthyroidism, hepatitis, TB and other deficiencies. This is from excessive nicotine, alcohol and drug abuse. Tobacco Mosiac virus (TVM) is another anxiety and depressive disorder found in humans. This is also found in the fetus that is caused by the use of tobacco products. You see, nicotine is the most (psychoactive) chemical in tobacco.

Nicotine increases dopamine inhibitors as it releases stress, alters mood and brain chemistry. Many individuals with psychiatric and anxiety disorders usually get fibromyalgia, diabetes and myalgia. This is usually passed on to the newborn. This is a cause of brain injuries and head injuries prior to the fetus becoming a newborn.

Finally, this is abortion. Abortion and miscarriage is a termination of pregnancy by the removal and or expulsion from the uterus of a fetus or embryo. In most cases, the pregnant individual may have psychological issues the warrants reason for termination of pregnancy. This can also be due to the negligence of the physician. However, in this day and age, I am being realistic. This is nonsense. Killing the head-fetus of anyone is ungodly and of Satan.

# PSYCHOSOCIAL AND MENTAL ILLNESS

Psychosocial relates to an individual's psychosocial development in interaction with social environment. This is that the individual's needs to fully understand and or comprehend the environment around him. Eric Erikson's stages of psychosocial development is flawed in various ways. Also, Robert Williams' Bitch, "Black Intelligence Test of Cognitive Homogeneity" and Ebonics are flawed. In addition, they are demonic and racist. They contain various forms, eight forms of misguidance. This misguidance has harmed millions of individuals from infancy to adulthood for decades.

2 Corinthians 2:11 In order that Satan might not outwit us for we are not unaware of his schemes and his satanic devices. Truly, these devices have aborted children mentally in the trillions for generations. And these are during this new era of education and psychiatry has delayed the development of everyone. This has made individuals commit crime and continue the murder while committing suicide. Throughout this scheme of things, we have lost our touch with reality.

In this, we have been filled with the anxieties of delusion, grandeur and social-comical arrogance. This pride is narcissistic and devious behavior which lacks both human and spiritual growth and development. This is the number one reason why the world has been tormented by evil forms of psychological practices. As I had written in my first book "Living Organisms", education is physiological. This means that our education system does not help in the proper mainstreaming and mediational aspects of spiritual and social learning. Neither does the church. They only seek to gain wealth through financial and mental gain.

They're of the Devil. They seek to steal, kill and destroy the soul of all unstable individuals that enter their establishment. This kind of thing must end. Let's begin teaching ourselves, embryos, children, adolescence, and other adults what is really going on. That is my receipt for success. We must present ourselves as babes when seeking a Godly knowledge. That is the only useful means of freedom and liberty.

Moving right along! In this, socialization means to become one the ones environment. To become an advocate for humanity by knowing his or her own destiny by not attempting to be a "holier than now" imbecile. Social interaction is to interact with others within ones current environment. This has nothing at all to do with any form of psychiatry. This is just the mercy of God. That is the deliverance of the people. In America, there is a freedom of love, honor and direction. This is within its' constitution. However, in many foreign nations the establishment of freedom is forever forbidden.

Now, in mental illness, individuals are often in denial of his or her own place. The individual then becomes delusional and narcissistic. Narcissism too is a mental disorder that is often difficult for the individual who is having this problem to notice. This is self-righteous. This often leads to a negative form of social behavior. This behavior is known as Heru-Tem Maat in the Khametic tradition and Raphael in the Caballistic tradition. These angels and deities then overpower the soul of the foolish and unstable.

Therefore, socialization and psychopathology relates to one understanding that God is the center of his or her life without exception. 2 Corinthians 4:3-4 there are some of whom the god of this age has blinded. The minds of the people. The spirit as a war against doctrines of demons.

Now, Erick Erickson's stages of development:

1. Hopes
2. Will
3. Purpose
4. Competence
5. Fidelity
6. Love
7. Care
8. Wisdom

Gives you a list of terms and age brackets defining what should happen once you get to a certain age. This is false prophecy. False prophecy leads to murder, abortions, hatred, homosexuality, covetousness and crime. This is written in Deuteronomy 18:1-22 and the entire book of Jude. Therefore, psychosocial as pertaining to socialization of the human genome and pathogens deal with adaptation and social behavior. Therefore, love thy neighbor as thy love thyself.

Now, in psychopathology that lies within mental illness. Mental illness such as bipolar, these individuals become extreme in areas of manipulation, have dormant behaviors and become easily angered. This is Sekert Tem Maat and Binah spirits of various eastern philosophies and religions. This is where individuals seclude themselves, become easily depressed, find themselves in darkness with anxiety. This is also where individuals do not function well in society. They are lazy and antisocial to some degree. They too are excessive alcoholics and drug abusers and are always looking for the sex-parties.

Also, in mental illness and social-dysfunctions as these individuals are often discussed in conversations as to having schemes within their within their conscious. Ivan Pavlov's theory of reflex and instinct has been another scheme within psychiatry. Of which it has denied humanity the understanding of their internal problems. Yet, he dealt with neurosciences. In this method Pavlov never discussed that individual had difficulties within the following areas of their lives; the PNS, CNS and ANS.

However, all areas deal with the internal nervous system as they assist the externalization of motor and cognitive development. You see, the spirit is above all things. Romans 1:30 tells us that negative things will be created by malicious individuals who are arrogant, boastful, slanderers, idolators and haters of God.

This leads to children being disobedient to parents. I can also say, they live in single parent homes or with a guardian. You see, this system fails the majority of time. This is due to the lack of education and poverty. Poverty often leads to no positive result. The results become vague. Vague to the point of one having to be institutionalized. This often leads to crime, murder and attempted suicide. Psychology is within the entire world is due to maladaptive behaviors, mental distress and having mental disorders.

This is then coined as abnormal psychology which is the study and field of medicine that studies abnormal patterns of behavior. Abnormal patterns of behavior are studied in non-western religions and cultures. In this, meditation is often used to trigger a certain behavior or spirit. Also, there are several forms and mechanisms of chanting that takes place. However;

The DSM-IV identifies three key elements that must be present to constitute a mental disorder. These elements include:

1. Symptoms that involve disturbances in behavior, thoughts and or emotions.
2. Symptoms that are associated with personal distress and or impairment.
3. Symptoms that stem from internal dysfunction; having biological and/or psychological roots.

The entire list above deals with negative functioning of the entire nervous system. The entire nervous system is a pathological existence of the brain. This is which leads every living organism to function within its environment properly. In this, mental illness is considered as being the number one disease of humankind. Everyone has a disorder.

Every illness is psychological. Therefore work with the spirit of God as education is physiological.